Dental School:
A Bizarre Comedy

D0880435

Acknowledgments

I wish to thank all those in my professional and personal lives who made this book possible.

Mr. Nick Productions, LLC

© 2015 by Mr. Nick Productions, LLC

Edited by my longtime friend and editor/writer,
Marilyn Milow Francis – Thank you!

Front and back covers – Jake Centofranchi
Book Layout – Jake Centofranchi

Photo of hapless dental school graduate – Anonymous
Published by Mr. Nick Productions, LLC © 2015

ISBN : 978-0-692-60806-7

0564

Dedications

To my father, who never once questioned my decision to attend dental school, and who gladly paid the tuition costs allowing me to become a "Doctor." And to my wife, who heard most of these "stories" as they unfolded. And to my children, who may get a chuckle out of them.

Foreword

Those four years in dental school weren't wasted, were they? They were the best four years of my life, right? It's hard to tell; it could have gone either way!

Although based on actual events, this is a book of humor and should be taken as such. There is no malicious intent; the only intent is to entertain!

Dr. I. Mayputz

TABLE OF CONTENTS

FRESHMAN YEAR

SOPHOMORE YEAR

JUNIOR YEAR

SENIOR YEAR

Introduction

This book is about a slightly fictionalized account of my life in dental school, inspired by actual events. Embellishments of strange happenings were unnecessary because human foibles ran rampant. However, all names and places have been changed so as not to embarrass the guilty, inept and downright scurvy. The stories are retold in a series of vignettes which best captured my mood at the time. These mostly bizarre and anguishing tales are set amidst a sea of often absurd and pressure-filled unrealistic expectations. But the heavy emotional carnage did have snippets of humor mixed in, which kept me relatively sane and enthusiastic. The end result was being called a Doctor! Was all the stress and aggravation worth it? The jury is still out as to whether I would have done it all over again.

Enjoy.

Dr. I. Mayputz

FRESHMAN YEAR

1

Fortuitous Party

This is how all the madness started. It was another rather innocuous but well attended third year pharmacy college party in the late '70s at my good friend D.'s apartment. All the regulars were already there. Even some girls showed up. After I arrived, things really *heated* up. I had a certain reputation in school. Fellow students didn't call me the Smallman for nothing. Suddenly there was smoke everywhere; it smelled like burned hemp. You know what I mean. Pharmacy students really knew how to *blow* off steam. Toward mid-night, after numerous shenanigans, like throwing a TV set out of a window, I chanced to bump into a former well-known student who had graduated that year. What he was doing at this soiree I'll never know. Anyway, we spoke briefly during our encounter. "What are you doing now, working for the family pharmacy business?," I yelled above the din. "No," he replied, "I'm a freshman in dental school." I asked, "Dental school, where?" He mumbled the location, it rhymed with Howard, but I didn't quite catch it.

That was it. Thirty seconds of chit chat that changed my life forever. I just didn't realize it at the time. A dentist. All the noise, debauchery and bullshit at that party seemed to fade in an instant. A dentist. This guy had made it to the next level. If he could do it, why not me? I stumbled home shortly thereafter in a smoky and drunken daze but that dental thought was already firmly implanted deep in my skull. A dentist. Good grief!

2

Fate or Tainted Luck?

I was working as a pharmacy intern in my future father-in-law's drugstore during the summer after my fourth year and still thinking about dental school. Yes or no? I needed some advice, some guidance, but from whom? In the coming fall I would be a senior at pharmacy college and had to get applications sent out, etc. Time was running out quickly. On an unusually slow day that summer, I was sent over to the local health center to hobnob with the physician, just for something to do and get some exposure to another medical field. I met the doctor and tried to socialize. He was seemingly bland but arrogant and "didn't have time for me," although there were no patients waiting. He dismissively suggested that maybe I should walk down the hall and meet "the dentist." So, I did just that. A kindly and gregarious man, he welcomed me with enthusiasm into his office. What a difference in medical demeanor! He was very busy with patients but asked if I wanted to observe. Fate, good fortune, neither? Whatever. I sat down in the assistant's chair and for the next few hours proceeded to avidly watch this guy drill, fill, extract, irradiate, mix, inject, etc. It was eye opening. I was actually excited, which was rare for me. I thanked him for the experience and literally ran back to the drugstore. I was thinking that I could do that kind of work. It looked easy. I believed that I could be even better than he, from what I had seen. My future father-in-law queried me about the physician but I went on and on about the dentist. It was beginning to become clear about what I should do in the fall: apply to dental school. And I did; however, as the school turned out to be, it wasn't as easy as I expected.

3

Applying

My mind was made up by the fall of my senior year of pharmacy college. I was going to be a dentist. Well, at least it sounded good. Now, about the application process. It would be easy, or so I thought. Senior year (fifth year in pharmacy college) was difficult, and here my thoughts were on dentistry. Our school had no post grad office or administrative officer to aid students in pursuits outside of pharmacy. Because no one could or would help me, I was directed to the library to help myself. The old and mean librarian (typical, although she wasn't an old maid) cackled loudly after I divulged my future plans to her and pointed with a gnarly index finger to a row of books on colleges. She walked away shaking her head and wringing her hands. Not a good sign. Hours were spent in that damn small library researching dental colleges, application procedures, dates, fees, etc. Although I figured out that I had enough time to apply, the Dental Admission Test (DAT) really concerned me. The next test would be in mid-October. It was now mid-September; no problem.

I drove my old, but trusty 1970 Plymouth Valiant (olive green color, what else) to a Barnes and Noble bookstore, purchased a Barron's DAT review book and cavalierly felt confident about life and my future. It was one of those beautiful sunny fall days when things looked like they would work out. I forgot, however, that Murphy lurked just around the corner ready to lay down his Law! It cost $35.00 to apply to five dental schools through a dental clearing house service. Why apply to any more? Five seemed about right (I found out later that most of my dental classmates had applied to at least twenty or thirty dental colleges under strict guidance by paid advisors). I was like the Fool in the major arcana of the Tarot: confident but careless. I picked schools that were in my geographically preferred area, sent in my $35.00 check and began studying in earnest for the DAT. Sure, I still had to get other stuff together– letters of recommendation, transcripts, personal letters, etc.– but the looming entrance test took precedence. It was only two weeks away! Fifth year pharmacy courses such as Medicinal Chemistry, Pharmaceutics II, Medical Therapeutics, Pharmaco-Kinetics II and Medicine lectures were tough going, but, I managed to study that Barron's review book as much as possible. I was going to be a dentist. After taking a few practice exams, it quickly dawned on me that I was either woefully unprepared or just plain dumb. Maybe, both. These practice tests were hard and I just wasn't scoring high enough to get in anywhere. Despair set in rather quickly. And, those damn pharmacy classes just kept getting tougher and tougher. It was senior year; give me a break, for God's sake! The DAT exam was set up in sections comprised of sciences, mathematics, three dimensional reckoning and reading comprehension. Similar to the SAT but harder. I just wasn't ready. I needed more time! I decided to skip the October exam and take it in April, at the application deadline. I read that most schools would still honor the April exam, although they preferred the previous October results. No one told me that in reality, the April results were basically for the following year, not the current one. Boy, was I naïve. I got all the application materials together, minus the DATs, and sent them out. I would take the DAT in April and be all set. What a moron. That's how I applied to dental school: on a whim and a prayer. If someone had told me at the beginning what my chances really were or how difficult it was to get a seat in dental college, I probably would not have bothered to apply. But, I did. I was going to be a dentist!

4

Dentist Wannabe

The application process was well underway. DATs (Dental Admission Test)? That's another story! I needed two letters of recommendation. I asked a close family friend back home (character witness, and boy was I a character, even back then) who just happened to be a college president. His daughter and I grew up together; as a child, I practically lived on his front porch in the summers. He really knew me. For the second letter, I figured I'd ask the dean/president of my locally well-known pharmacy college, where I was currently a senior. Why not have two big fish write letters for me? I needed all the help I could get! Even I knew that much. My undergrad college was small; everyone knew everyone, and their business! Of course, the dean knew me personally, or at least it seemed that way whenever we passed each other in the school's hallways. He was a very short, stout, gruff, unfunny and decent man. Very old school. I was granted an audience with him after scheduling an appointment with his brusque secretary. Well, she wasn't really mean, just overly and needlessly professional. As I entered his immaculate office, he peered up at me from behind his desk while scanning my transcripts, and in a gravelly voice said, "So, you want to be a dentist, do you?" How did he know? Only my roommate and girlfriend knew, or so I thought. Someone had narked, but I wasn't surprised. Anyway, he shook his head gravely while reading those damn grades of mine. It wasn't a good sign. I meekly sat down across from him and asked if he could see his way clear and write a letter on my behalf. Silence. He pondered that question, scratched his balding pate and removed his Coke-bottle thick glasses. Very sternly, he finally blurted out, "We'll say in the letter that you were in the top 1/3 of your class! It should help get you in." I was so happy. The president of my college was actually going to stick his neck out and help the class joker. What a guy! But why would he help me, an insignificant peon at the school? I was well known, but not for any scholarly endeavors. Was my B plus average really that good; good enough for dental school? Well, I thanked him up and down as I vigorously shook his hand and prepared to leave when he suddenly told me to sit back down. He had a story to relate to me. What story? He now seemed a bit angry and spaced out. Uh oh! He proceeded to spin a woeful tale of also wanting to become a dentist. Who knew? After graduating from pharmacy college he got as far as the second year in a very prestigious Midwestern dental college. At the beginning of his second year he received a dreaded letter, which he showed me, that bluntly outlined his "ineptitude" in the laboratory portions of his studies. You know, the parts that involve eye-hand coordination and three dimensional visualizations. Apparently, he just couldn't cut it (pun intended)! The letter, signed by the president of the dental school, ended with his dismissal. It was official, alright. I just sat there squirming in my seat. Awkward. My president still seemed bitter after all these years. Silence, again. He finally spoke and implored me to do better than he had done, to show "those bastards" that a pharmacy college grad could "cut the mustard," as he put it. I guessed my acceptance would be sweet vindication for him. However, it would still be a tough road ahead for me, especially without any advisory guidance. His mood brightened somewhat as he reverently stowed away that "sacred" letter of failure and started to talk tennis to me. It turned out that he was a nationally ranked player in the over 75's category. Who knew? And, who knew that he was actually a dental school dropout? His secret was safe with me. After he was canned from dental school, he proceeded to obtain his Ph.D. in pharmacy, began teaching and finally became dean/president of my college. I eventually did write him (before email, texts or cellphones) upon my graduation as a dentist. He wrote back a one sentence reply– "You did it for all of us." I guess I did. A little belated payback to the dental gods? I still have his one sentence letter, safely tucked away, somewhere.

5

The Dreaded DAT

No one likes standardized tests, well, at least I don't. One
of my children does; he's an extraordinarily gifted mammal,
however. Anyway, after studying on my own for months,
I felt I was somewhat ready to take that dreaded dental
entrance exam and get on with my life. I still wanted to be a
dentist! I had sent my DAT application fee in earlier by snail
mail (that's all we had back then, no online anything), and
was set to take it at a large university in my town. I heard
absolutely nothing from the five schools I had applied to
and hoped that they indeed had received all my application
materials. I guess I could have called to confirm things, but
didn't. The day arrived and I was more than nervous. My
girlfriend tried her best to calm me down. It was no use.
I had gotten better on the practice tests but still needed
to improve. And, the three-dimensional parts were mind
numbing. It was bullfuck! I got into my trusty Plymouth
Valiant, waved goodbye to my future wife, and drove slowly
and deliberately to the testing site. People assumed I was an

old lady driving that car; nobody honked or seemed pissed off while passing me. The running joke in the '80s was that many little old ladies drove Plymouth Valiants. With my methodical and slow driving habits, I fit right in. I really didn't know where I was going. No GPS, no specific driving directions, just a general idea where the university was. It was a Saturday. I managed to find the place and a parking spot and proceeded to enter the wrong building. Hey, they all looked the same to me. Because it was a Saturday, there were very few students milling around on campus. I had just five minutes to get to the test and there was no one to ask for directions. And, I had to pee. Finally, someone appeared exiting from a nearby dorm and I launched myself at that person. She recoiled at my boldness and told me where to go, but gave me accurate directions as well. I made it in time– to a bathroom– and then found a seat with no time to spare. I was sweating bullets as I looked around the large classroom. It was filled to capacity with about 200 would-be dental students, all serious looking and ready. Was I ready? I had my #2 pencils and they were sharpened! Before we started, there was the mandatory check of students with ID that matched the test, the obligatory pre-testing speeches by the proctors, and the announcement that the soap and knife portion had been discontinued. What? The what soap and what knife portion? All the other students exhaled sighs of relief. I exhaled, period. It turns out that all previous exams had a special part where testees (I like that word) were handed a bar of soap, a tooth figurine, a short lab knife, and instructed to carve the soap as best as possible in the allotted time to resemble the fake tooth model in front of them. And, no do-overs. Instead of this manual dexterity test, there would be an additional three-dimensional examination part on the test. I was always good at carving things and gluing models together. I might have carved quite a tooth out of that bar of soap. Little did I know that during first year of dental school, carving and modeling wax shapes were required ad nauseam. I would get my chance and then some to whittle, chisel, and mold to the nth degree. The exam commenced and, five hours later, thankfully ended. It went okay. Some parts were actually similar to the practice tests I had taken. Reading comprehension was about pharmacy problems, which I hoped I aced. I found out later in the foyer outside the classroom that most, if not all of the students, had diligently and professionally prepared for the exam by taking a Stanley Kaplan prep course or equivalent. I had heard of him. But it never occurred to me to take a prep course. Idiot! I received the results about a week later. Overall, I scored an average of five on a scale of one-to-nine. Just average, according to the adjoining graph in the results packet. I got a nine as expected on the reading comp. part. Maybe that score would get me in, or at least get me noticed. All five dental schools acknowledged receipt of said scores. Now, I waited.

6

The Interview— What the F...?

I only told my parental units about dental school after I received an interview invite from PU College of Dentistry in late April of my senior year, just after I took the DAT entrance exam. Why build up hopes when you don't have to? I was frosted by the other four dental schools I had applied to; no interviews, no nothing. Although, the University of Buffalo said I would be considered for its class the following year. Would be considered was not the same as an interview and/or admission. Plus, I didn't want to shuffle off to Buffalo and be so far away from my soon-to-be fiancée. My parents had a dumbstruck reaction to my deadpan delivered news. Dental school? All kinds of inane questions just kept pouring out of that phone receiver. That's why I hesitated to tell them in the first place. My father stated the obvious when he asked, "How the hell did you get in with such bad grades?" Well, I retorted that this was just the interview, and my grades placed me in the top third of my class— just barely. Mom and Dad were old-fashioned, somber, and highly educated college professors and they understood higher education. Maybe that's why they were so confused over my news. Only "those" kids got into medical and dental schools. How did I manage such a coup? I wasn't special, a "brainiac," or connected. But, apparently this college wanted me, for some reason. Pop finally did say that he was willing to shell out big bucks if I was really going to become a "Doctor." His consternation quickly turned to elation about my new career choice. It suddenly became important to him and for the family bragging rights. That's right: a doctor in the house! I had to remind everyone that this was the interview, I wasn't admitted yet. However, it was good to hear enthusiastic people around me for a change. Even my very reserved and stoic mother was giddy with pride. My father took a day off to drive me to the interview. He knew the town well from past educational experiences there and knew right where to go. The four hour trip was filled with small talk– no mention of the pharmacy college courses I had received Cs in, or my girlfriend, or other hot button subjects. I think he had new respect for me. Maybe? He double-parked next to the "dental" building, wished me well, and waited in the car as I disappeared inside. The security guard in the foyer took my name, gave me a temporary "official" badge, and escorted me to the elevator banks (there were four giant elevators) with directions to the interview room. I distinctly remembered this friendly guard with a thick Hispanic accent; we would meet again, soon. Many white-coated students milled about in the lobby and in front of the elevators as if in an asylum. I wanted to be a part of this lunacy; I just knew. I entered the "interview room" and sat down in the on-deck circle amidst a panoply of smug-looking, sharply dressed interviewees. Some were already finished and kibitzing, some were cockily bantering out loud. Was this display nervous bravado or were these jerks potential future classmates? Alas, you already know the answer. My name was finally called and just as I went through to the actual interview room I clearly overheard someone in that waiting room mention that he took the Stanley Kaplan interview prep course. Stanley again? What interview prep course? Boy, did I suddenly feel unprepared. This was not going to go well, and it didn't. I was already edgy from the long drive, the long wait and the Stanley Kaplan comment. However, it was my turn to be grilled, and brother was I barbecued! I sat down in front of two very dour-looking professors; one, the biochemistry chairwoman and dean of admissions, and the other, a "beloved" and long-tenured biochemistry professor. Why biochemistry professors and not dental professors (actual dentists)? I don't know. Well, both of them let loose on me like two untethered pit bulls. One blatantly accused me of wasting their time with my "low" grades, the other accused me of taking a spot away from an actual bio major because I already had a professional career (pharmacy). One demanded to know why

I had two college presidents write recommendation letters? Weren't "lowly" professors good enough for me? This barrage of insulting questions continued unabated with only shrugs, nods and grunts from me. Finally, after another low blow, I spoke up. Big mistake. I rebutted every previous insult with a defensive remark and backed up every retort with logical reasoning, or so I reckoned. Well, my reckoning only made them more incensed. We three had a free-wheeling shouting match going on before I calmed down and stepped off.

The last question shot at me was to identify– if I could– a butterfly from an insect book on their desk. I had mentioned in my application that I was an amateur naturalist/entomologist. Now I had to prove it! I got lucky. The butterfly was a common male Monarch butterfly and I easily and correctly identified it, much to their chagrin. I was then testily and brusquely asked to vacate the premises at once. I knew where I was not wanted, but this school did send me an interview request, hadn't it? I was confused and dejected. I had failed and felt miserable. It was way too late for Stanley Kaplan to rescue me. But then, out of nowhere, the portly biochemistry chairwoman scuttled after me and beckoned me to her private lair. I was hot, sweaty and angry, but followed her, all the while being stared at by the other hapless students-in-waiting. She closed the door and glared at me. Was this going to be more punishment, piling on? What did I ever do to her? She bluntly asked me how I took notes, how I studied, why I really wanted to be a dentist? In restrained, measured tones, I answered as best I could. She seemed to like what she heard from me. After a few minutes, she ushered me out, smiling that "knowing" grin at me. I guess she liked my act after all. I don't know if any other potential dental student got the Part II interview from her. Was I that good, was I the only sap with the audacity to fire back when fired upon, or were they desperate for my father's moola? Maybe two out of three? This had been my only dental school interview thus far. No one else seemed to want me. I remained cautiously hopeful, regardless of the tumultuous interview ministrations that had just transpired. My father had been waiting patiently, still double-parked, for approximately two hours. He remarked at my slovenly appearance. I quietly told him that I had been beaten up, both literally and figuratively. We left the dental town. No questions were asked, no answers would have been given. I was wiped out. I slept all the way home. Hopefully the madhouse I had just left would come through because I was insanely ready to be a dentist!

7

The Waiting Game

I had already thrown out the DAT review book. And I already had my first interview with a dental school. Pharmacy college was winding down and I was eager and ready for more interviews and possible admittance. I waited, and waited some more. It was now getting close to pharmacy board exams and graduation. It was now or never. Then, three rejection letters in two days had me depressed. All three commented that they could not seriously consider me because I had taken the DAT too late for entry that year, and all available seats were taken. The fourth school replied that it would consider me as an applicant for the following year if I chose to reapply. I could either use my current DAT scores or retake the exam. I wasn't promised admission but strongly advised to reapply. I was now 0 for 4 with one school to go. Meanwhile, I had a verbal agreement with Rite Aid Pharmacy to work for it in my home town. My parents were very happy; local boy makes good and comes home. Or, should I say "loco" boy! They didn't bring up the subject of dentistry at all, as if it was a non starter. My girlfriend was saddened not only for me but for the prospect of her possibly moving to my home town and living close to my parents. Plus what would she do when she graduated from pharmacy college? My town only had one pharmacy. May 15th, a Saturday, dawned early, and we slept in. By noon my girlfriend woke up and went to get the mail. She came back and looked unhappy while handing me a letter. Her downcast look said it all. She held a white paper in her hand and had obviously read it. I snatched it from her and then yelled a profanity out loud. The school that had granted me the lone interview had accepted me. Period. I could have killed her for purposely teasing me. We made up rather quickly, and her smile returned. Well, not too quickly. Finally, it was time to be a dentist! I couldn't help rereading that fateful letter over and over again. The first call went to my father. There was silence on the other end, then weak congratulations. How did *he* get in? This kind of thing only happened to those *other* brainy or connected kids. At least my mom sounded glad, sort of. (They had both been excited by my interview but then realized my slim-to-none chances of actually getting in. So, they played down my prospects as a dentist and were literally shocked at my acceptance.) Rite Aid got the brush off next. Call upon call was made until I couldn't think of anyone else to contact. My roommate came by in the afternoon to announce that he was accepted the day before to a Ph.D. program in medicinal chemistry at a prestigious college down south. Two of the biggest partyers and eccentrics in the class were moving on up in life. Who would have figured that? Of course, we three celebrated with some rare "Hawaiian" herb. My girlfriend was happy but sad that I would be far away from her for at least two years, until she graduated. I could tell by the look on her face that all of a sudden, she was uncertain of the future. Maybe living in my hometown didn't sound like a bad idea after all. It was a heady time, with finals, pharmacy board exams, graduation and dental thoughts all jumbled together. I don't know how I passed everything, but I did. It was now late June, my girlfriend was working at the VA hospital as a pharmacy intern and I was back home working as a pharmacist in a small pharmacy in an adjacent town, just for the summer. My mind was squarely focused on dental school, and on one more thought. In July I did the right thing by surprising my girlfriend with a visit and made her my fiancée. For a nonchalant type of tough mountain girl, she melted a bit. Phone calls burst forth and friends were made to look at that rock on her finger. She was going to be a "doctor's" wife. None of this had been in our future plans when we first started dating and mating. None of it. We were going to be pharmacists and that's it. This dental thing was either going to be a curse or a blessing. But, I had to take the chance. Everyone gets opportunities in life, and some actually act on them. This was my moment. *Carpe diem.* What's the worst that could happen? I could fail out, my father would lose the tuition money, and I would be a Rite Aid pharmacist. A bad loss, but not that bad. However, if I made it, maybe someday I could own a beachfront villa on some island in the Bahamas. That's how I thought back then. Was it all worth it? It's hard to tell. I did make it through dental school (summa cum laude) and we do own a beachfront villa on an island called GHC, in the Bahamas. You tell me.

8

Old Doc Smithe

I had recently been accepted to a dental school and was home, working my summer job as a pharmacist in a neighboring village. My folks liked having me home, at least for the three months that I would be there. I was still in a state of euphoria and considered myself a dental-student-in-waiting. Sort of like being in the on-deck circle in baseball. Driving by his house/practice on Main Street, I spied old Doc Smithe sitting in the proverbial rocker on his front porch, looking thin and frail in the evening sunlight. He had been our crabby small town dentist for years and years when I was growing up. In his prime, in the 1940s, he had been the "cat's meow." It was widely known that he was the first dentist in our county to procure and use x-ray equipment, the first to do "therapeutic cleanings," etc. I remember him having few bedside manners and being rather callous with my sister and me. Maybe he disliked kids? He was the only act in town for decades and, along with "Digger" the undertaker, was a necessary evil. Now, he was long retired, very old, ill, and basically forgotten. He was obsolete! I parked my car and excitedly bounded up his porch steps to tell him my news. "Hi Doc, I got into dental school. I'm going to PU," I shouted out loudly. He just stared straight ahead, stone-faced, not making any eye contact. Maybe he was too ill to reply. I just stood there, awkwardly, waiting for a positive response. Finally, he cleared his throat and gruffly retorted, "I went to Penn." And, that was it. No further verbiage was uttered. He proceeded to dismissively wave me off his porch and I gingerly stepped away, slowly, like backing away from a rattlesnake. I was angry that day and harbored that anger for many years hence. He really pissed me off. What could have been a joyous and celebratory encounter never materialized. I was looking for a nod of approval from a doctor I respected. I thought he would welcome me to the "Dental Club." He did not. Was it his illness and infirmity, his Ivy snobbery (Penn is an Ivy League college, PU is not), a lifetime of disappointments and disillusionment? All of the above? What soured him? I don't know. However, as I reflect on my own looming retirement, I can at least empathize with him a bit. Will I be crabby some day? Will I grumpily chase a prospective dental student off my stoop in my old age? Maybe old Doc Smithe suffered more than any of us realized, or perhaps he was just an elitist, Ivy-educated, pompous prick who thought we country bumpkins were way beneath him. I'll never know for sure. I know I should let it go, but that "Penn" comment still chafes me.

9

Living Derangements

In the four years of dental college, I lived in four disparate parts of town, in four unique domiciles. Each had its own "charm," which I'm sure was mostly lost on me. Back then, especially during the first two years, I was concerned with dental learning, food and shelter; kind of like a Neanderthal with books. The four separate moves involved my parents. Although stressful, I greatly appreciated their help each time. First year, I was without my wife; she was still my fiancée, more than four hours away. It had been a major debacle getting a place to live. Numerous phone calls during the summer with prospective student roommates and even a visit proved fruitless. Finally, I received a friendly call from a witty duffer who was from the city, but did *not* want to live at home and commute to the dental college. He had gotten my name from the "desperate section" of the dental school housing bulletin board. He wanted to split a small apartment with a roommate. Great, someone wanted to live with me besides my fiancée! He boastfully claimed to have lots of leads, but they all fizzled, one by one. And time ticked by. I had, however, to believe in him. What else could I do because the school was of no help to me whatsoever? When I questioned the college about the possibility of living in its limited dorm space, I was instantly shot down. Why? I lived more than four hours away. Surely I was a good candidate for housing? More about that later; I'm still frosted over it, hence no alumni donations! "They" told me to keep trying. Keep trying to do what? Magically conjure up living accommodations? Dental anxiety was not just for patients. It started early for me, and needlessly. I had heard whispers that PU College of Dentistry was the school of hard knocks, and it was fast proving it. My potential roommate and I started to feel desperate as the days went by. Daily phone calls to each other reflected our nervous tension. At least he could live at home and commute in; what was I to do, live in the bus station and sleep on a bench? My parents really didn't know how to help me so they were out of the loop. A week before school started, I frantically phoned him and he excitedly reassured me that we would be living temporarily at his girlfriend's one bedroom apartment, for cheap rent, in a seedy part of town. He obviously had felt compelled to help me. His ego and promises wouldn't let me down, thank goodness. And, a witless dental student from Kennebunkport would also be joining us as a roommate. Great! Did his *shiksa* girlfriend know that the circus was coming to her pad? An apartment with a teeny living room, a puny fridge, an itsy-bitsy oven, and an even smaller bathroom? I don't think she knew at all about the living arrangements. On the morning we three moved in, she just kept staring at us and her boyfriend, back and forth. She spoke very little that day. The move was difficult and sweaty. My parents dutifully and silently unloaded me and my meager belongings. My bed was the living room sofa; my blanket, the couch comforter. The guy from Maine brought a fold-out portable bed that he planted next to the couch. No desks, no closets, no privacy, and only one lavatory. My Mom just rolled her eyes. My father was happy; I was enrolled, period. That's how I started dental school. The living accommodations were sparse and crude, the conditions were deplorable and the atmosphere tense. The floor instantly became littered with dental wax shavings and plastic and real teeth, as all three of us attempted to study and learn at home. The girlfriend was quietly freaking out as September dragged into October. I tried to stay at school as long as possible and get as much work done as I could there. I liked the girlfriend and was grateful for her unplanned hospitality. However, it was a twenty minute trek home, in the dark, in a very bad part of town. But, I did it; I walked home many times, late at night to help preserve her sanity. I don't remember doing laundry, washing the dishes, taking a shower or cleaning the bathroom. It's funny what you don't recall when traumatized! This unfulfilling ménage à trois plus one, crammed into a pocket-sized hole-in-the-wall rental, came to a blissful end at the end of October. We found a very large, one bedroom apartment in a better part of town, and closer to the dental college. The rent was steeper, although I did get my own bed! We moved again. My mom and dad eagerly helped me this time. All smiles, all around. The beleaguered girlfriend was all smiles, too. Those pungent scents of unwelcome dental materials combined with the stench of nervous male sweat would finally be gone from her apartment. The rest of my housing history lurched and crept forward over the years. Private lodgings morphed into dental dorm living, followed by private digs once more. Moving multiple times was a pain in the ass. My roommates and I split up after first year, as did the duffer and his girlfriend. The Irish dude from Kennebunkport decided to split, permanently. He evidently hated dentistry and had been doing abysmally academically. Most of my classmates were then astonished to learn that he ended up attending a medical school somewhere in the Caribbean. A dolt who couldn't cut his way around a tooth probably turned into a doctor, after all! Good Lord! The original boastful duffer (who was previously a bartender in town) was also annoyingly intelligent and determined, and rose up to be the four-year class president and valedictorian of our class. Good Lord!

10

Welcome!

The morning air was crisp and everyone was up and bustling around. You could hear the endless taxi bleatings in the distance. Everything seemed brand new to me: the living arrangements, my roomies, the very sidewalk. I was excited, which was rather unusual for me. Never mind the extremely cramped, one bedroom third story apartment I shared with two fellow freshmen dental students and the rightful tenant– one of my roommate's girlfriend. Ah, the first day of school. What a headrush feeling. That first morning we pushed past a grumbling and disheveled girlfriend and took the building elevator to the lobby. Black was the motif in the building: black speckled flooring, black paneling, and black granite columns with white accents. It was a rather swanky building in a dilapidated part of town, but I wouldn't have called it posh. As we three wiseguys bantered nervously on our way toward school, I noticed what seemed like a large object perched atop a storm drain grate next to the curb. One roommate nonchalantly walked around it. Another stepped over it. I stopped and stared. An old "bag lady" (the word "homeless" was not yet in vogue) was squatting over the grate and urinating in broad daylight. She had on the requisite battered, and slimed-up attire complete with gnarly-looking flats on her feet. If it had been Halloween, the outfit would have been appropriate. But in September? Anyway, she cocked her head sideways, raised a dirty clawed hand and flipped me off before snarling, "Welcome home, boyfriend!" Welcome, indeed. Did my newness really show that much? Any naiveté on my part quickly dissipated after that incident. My introduction to the really have-nots was serendipitous but had a profound effect on me because I still remembered it all these years later. Was that empathy I was feeling? Maybe dentistry was the right field for me. Maybe?

11

What's in a Name?

First day of classes. We were all gathered in the school's largest auditorium for a morning meet-and-greet session. Showered, lab coats on, name tags affixed, we ventured forth into the fray. There were professors present, coffee, doughnuts and most important, about 140 wide-eyed and tremulous freshmen. What a motley assemblage! So, as I began chatting with a bunch of guys I would never befriend or even give the time of day to, names came up. The required name tags revealed many ethnic, original surnames. Interestingly, there were no typical American names such as Jones, Smith, Black, White or Brown. Where did *they* all go to college? Anyway, Richard Hertz introduced himself as a wealthy musician from Long Island, whose father was also a dentist. I asked him if I could call him Dick. He glared at me in confusion. Hadn't anyone ever called him Dick before? Was he that rich that even his butler had to call him Richard? The group didn't get the joke, either. Dick-Hertz? Get it? Crickets from the audience! Corny but still mildly amusing, I mistakenly thought. This was going to be a tough crowd and a tough year. Those guys already seemed to be uptight "doctors" and in no mood for sophomoric cornball comedy. Nevertheless, they started calling me Izzy, not Isadore, or even Isaac. Izzy? I hadn't been called that since 6th grade. But it wasn't an insult. Curiously, William asked to be called Billy; Daniel insisted on being called Danny. Maybe it was a city thing or a sign of familiarity. I don't know. Or, a wealthy and privileged thing, like women being called Poppy, Buffy or Tipper. I was now Izzy, again. No nicknames. At least they got my last name right on the first try. Back in college, no one attempted to pronounce my last name or try to spell it. No problem here; and no one asked me my nationality or "where I was from" either. Not even the professors. I was thrown into a scalding melting pot called dental school stew and was glad of it. I was grateful and felt like I finally belonged. Except, of course, for being called Izzy!

12

Student Body and Mind

Although I fancied myself a reasonably intelligent and attractive man with a decent physique (after all, I did manage to attract my hottie blondie fiancée), I was nonetheless anxious about stacking up to "really serious" professional school students. They were all probably smarter and better looking than I. Boy, I was never more wrong. What a mix of misshapen and intellectually stunted people. Not everyone, mind you, but the vast majority fit into that ragtag rubric. My cursory glance at the freshmen class revealed an array of unattractive females and gorky, dorky males. What is it with professional schools and ugly student bodies? It's not just hearsay. I was there! I witnessed the fugly! Although sexist to say, when our school's lone attractive female graced our hallways, guys stood still and stared. Time stood still. It was that rare of a sight. Besides being mostly physically unfit and unkempt, the mental prowess and wits of my fellow students were often called out by me. Here I was, from "Bumfuck," N.Y., having more sense and guile than those "worldly" urbanites. I was prepared to be eaten up by this so-called savvy crowd. Instead, I ended up running roughshod on these "dumbasses" as evidenced after the first few exams. Although I did have an edge already being a pharmacist, there was no excuse for their lack of mental acuity. And this was the cream of the crop, in dental school? Of course, these same students blindly and arrogantly prided themselves as being "cool" and "all that." I was always astonished by the sheer willpower of some students, even in the face of obvious ineptitude. I had mistakenly thought that I would finally meet my match with some other smart, wise-cracking types, maybe even forge a friendship or two. No dice, at first. Many after school parties involved infantile drinking games, '80s music (of course, this was the '80s) and no monkey business. One time I produced a pin joint of Panama Red from behind my ear and nearly emptied the place. I wasn't going to turn the place into an opium den, honest! Another time a bit of laced Hash in a hash pipe elicited panic and almost got me kicked out from a paltry party. Hell, in college, many parties didn't actually start until I arrived. Even my girlfriend in college (whom I married) first knew me by my "illicit" reputation. Here, in dental school, I was a degenerate? Not really, though. Even in pharmacy college I was an aficionado, a lightweight smoker, not a hard core stoner as imagined by my peers. I knew my limits and was a devoted student. My reputation while there was often a victim of hype rather than fact. Of course, I never sought to quell the rumors and actually reveled in the notoriety. I did manage, however, to barely acquaint myself with a few like minded souls in my freshman dental journey. And, once my wife joined me, I finally had a co-conspirator and best friend I could relate to. Very few of my fellow dental students realized just how much and how diligently I studied the dental craft and eventually were amazed to discover my high class rank at graduation. But I kept true to myself throughout; joking, brow-beating, and good-naturedly insulting all comers. Once a clown, always a clown.

13

"Effeminate Chic"

What was it about some of my male dental school colleagues, especially the rich city kids? I know it was the "crazy" eighties, but still, what was up? In undergrad, men were men, women were... Here, in dental school, the lines were blurred just a bit. What was this effeminate subculture among these men? They weren't gay, at least not to my knowledge, or their girlfriends. Were they homosexual wannabes? The attire, the mannerisms, the excess jewelry, etc., made these "boys" appear androgynous and metrosexual to me. Was it on purpose or just an eighties fad? I didn't understand these affectations. Of course, being somewhat of a hick, I never read GQ magazine or had even heard of Perry Ellis. Maybe I was confusing haute couture and Emily Post manners with transgender tendencies? Conversely, the professional women of those days seemed to be going in the "masculine" direction– pantsuits without cleavage potential, little or no jewelry, no-heel flats, and short bobs on their heads. Meanwhile, big hair, bare and hairy chests, and faux feminism were becoming popular with "manly" rock stars like the *bois* of Twisted Sister. It was all so ambiguous and mixed up. The eighties, I'm glad, are so over!

14

Freshmen Teeth?

I received a curious memo from PU College of Dentistry in the summer prior to starting classes, mandating students to bring extracted teeth with them to school. However, it made perfect sense. After all, *this was dental school!* The memo did not specify the amount of teeth necessary or which ones, for that matter. I dutifully dropped off two small jars at two separate local offices I called upon, and the dentists there were happy to oblige my request. I was all set for school. Wrong! Imagine my shock and awe upon seeing the huge glass gallon containers that most other freshmen pulled out from backpacks in our first laboratory sessions. Those jars were absolutely bursting with teeth– hundreds and hundreds of them. Containers full of teeth graced the laboratory bench tops as far as the eye could see. I pulled out two small Mason jars with a measly total of seven teeth! I didn't know *that* many cuspids and premolars were needed. I didn't know that I should have dropped a jar off at an oral surgeon's office and not a general dentist's practice. I got the memo but it was not specific. Those extracted teeth would be set up in artificial jaws and worked upon. That's how we started learning; drill and fill, baby! Well, I got my quota of molars by begging and borrowing from others' vast stashes. Talk about high anxiety. But I wasn't the only naïve one around; some students started with no teeth at all. Somehow, we all learned to share, sometimes begrudgingly, and we got through those trying first year labs. It was nerve wracking and pressure filled. Just another example of the duress put upon us by the school, and we had just begun! Nevertheless, we cut, drilled, filled, polished and moved on– to *more* unjustified aggravation, all in the name of dental education.

15

Fool's Gold

The entire class was duly lectured ad nauseam during the first week of school *not* to extract gold fillings or gold crowns from the cadavers and then sell them to merchants in the town's "gold district." Simple and contrite orders that even a dummy could understand. Not so fast, however. Evidently the advice fell on deaf, dummy ears. During each prior year, several students were expelled for doing some illegal "gold digging." Our year was no exception. A trap was set; the sting successful. Our class became lighter by five students after just two weeks of school. All that wasted studying and preparation to get in. All that embarrassment on getting booted out. What else can I say?

16

A Real Mensch

One of my first laboratory experiences was with Dental Materials Science, a lab designed to acquaint the freshman dental student with all the materials used in dentistry (circa 1980s, of course). We were seated alphabetically in rows of ten, each behind black colored, marble-topped work benches complete with every bell, whistle and gizmo attachment. A handyman would have felt right at home working at a bench like that. The lab's department head and lead professor was highly respected, personable, and strictly observant (Lubavitch Orthodox). His calm and reassuring demeanor gave us greenhorns solace as we unpacked large fishing tackle boxes full of strange looking stuff! No worries though, each lab session started off with a short film describing the necessary armamentarium (I hate that word) and protocols of usage. We diligently followed along in the lab manual as well. Couldn't be easier, right? Wrong! After all, we were beginners at this thing called "dental school." "Today, we are going to learn how to solder gold," he remarked. "Please put on your protective eyewear." I thought, "Are you kidding me?" I looked around the room and saw panic on most students' faces. Soldering? At least I had some prior experience, having learned arc welding in seventh and eighth grade metal shop at my high school. It was a mandatory course for all boys at my school at the time. At my rural high school, many of the graduates returned to farming, animal husbandry, etc. Welding was just a necessity of the area. When I spoke up that I knew how to light an acetylene torch, my row mates recoiled from me in horror. This "redneck" from "Bumfuck," N.Y., with the wide "bulletproof" ties (thin ties were all the rage in the '80s) knew how to solder? It made sense! In walked our row instructor at last. Short, large glasses, with a gait similar to Groucho Marx and a face like Woody Allen. He also had that rumpled Columbo (Peter Falk) look about him. Friday afternoon and he was done with his private patients; he was here to unwind, pick up a few bucks, and maybe stroke his ego by teaching us lowlifes something. He had his swanky briefcase slung over his back with a squash racket sticking out of it (he didn't actually play; it was a male status symbol at the time). He sat down, unprepared, and hurriedly checked out the neighboring rows to see what they were doing. After name introductions and much hesitation, we began. It was easy for me, having handled soldering equipment and torches before. It was like getting back on a bike; you never forget. Because I seemed adept at this initial foray into dentistry, our instructor naturally gravitated to me. Peering closely at my work, he would sometimes remove his glasses, lick them front and back, and wipe them with his narrow tie. So much for cross-contamination. But I liked this guy. There was something about him and his down to earth work ethic that resonated with me. Other students blew him off as a flaky character. I bonded with him, instead. Well, during the rest of the year, everything I did appeared golden to him. Actually it was, at least compared to the bumblers in my row! This pattern continued for the length of the course; I received the only "honors" grade in my row. This instructor asked me numerous times if I desired a part-time job after school at his office. I said "no" as a freshman but took him up on it during third year. And, I'm glad I did.

17

Neatness Counts

You would walk into the back of a dental laboratory and see students from different years furiously scrubbing, washing and polishing stone models and cursing loudly; mainly the women, mind you. It was always amusing to witness demure and normally reserved women, *of the opposite sex,* launch into tirades of unprovoked profanity. That's what dental school did to you. It lowered inhibitions at inopportune times! Neatness counted, big time. Why? Well, you didn't want to go to a sloppy, messy and disheveled dentist, did you? So, the rigorous "re-education" and training of us bozos started early, in freshman year, actually on the first day of class! You had to quickly develop a certain self-awareness and religiously clean up after yourself. Sounds New Age, doesn't it? If you were born a meticulous and fastidious person, you were golden in dental school; if you weren't, things could get ugly in a hurry. All grades received for observed and handed-in work included an "unwritten" neatness mark. Neatness mark? Yes, that's right, it was factored into your final grade in all that you did.

This neatnik paradigm pervaded the entire school, all classes, and only compounded the already highly charged and tense atmosphere of learning dentistry, in general. Performing under pressure while neatly maintaining composure and tidiness were the hallmarks to be aspired to. Obviously, some students fared better than others. Those who had a modicum of eye-hand coordination and had dexterously used their hands while growing up seemed more adept in the neatness department. Maybe all those plastic model cars and planes I glued together as a kid weren't such a waste of time after all, although, sniffing the glue could have altered my pea-brain a bit. Maybe that's why I decided on dentistry as a career choice; the acetone and toluene glue vapors could have been responsible for subtly influencing me. Of course, the open containers of worm wood oil, benzene and chloroform inside malfunctioning laminar flow hoods in pharmacy college may have further damaged my gray matter as well. That may explain my "addled" cognitive state during my dental school decision making process. It all makes sense now. Hey, at least I'm a neatnik. Yay!

18

Biochemistry Blues

Very few freshmen had previously taken biochemistry in college. Most, if not all, had heard that it was a tough course. But I had taken it in pharmacy college, complete with a strenuous lab. I struggled with it then and managed to eke out a low B. The dental school laboratory portion proved to be relatively easy for me; it was a watered down repeat of my previous lab experiences. Anyhow, the class portion was a nightmare. We started with simple sugars, like glucose, fructose, galactose, etc. The gratuitous and seemingly funny and friendly lead professor implored us not to memorize anything in class, just get the basic ideas. It sounded reasonable. He was a dynamic lecturer and convincing prophet of "easy" science. My fellow students actually believed him. I had a previous run-in with him during my interview. I didn't like him! His classroom theatrics of reducing complicated biochemical processes and reactions to simple ideas were appalling to me. I knew better; I had been through this hell before. I told my peers loudly and forcefully outside of class not to buy in to his bullshit. Sure enough, the first exam straightened us all out. Suffice it to say that even after valiant study, I managed to get an 80, with a 40 point curve! The class president (my freshman roommate and future valedictorian) only mustered an 81. The exam had required us to write out the complete Kreb's cycle, Pyruvic Acid cycle, etc., etc. All stuff that we were told NOT to memorize. I guess if you were a biochemistry major or wizard, you could have figured all of this out during the exam. We were just lowly dental students in first year. Well, most students did so poorly as to elicit a response from the college president. He and the Biochemistry department staff called us the dumbest class ever to crawl through the hallowed halls of our dental school. There were calls for us to start the year over, or maybe take the course again as second year students. Remember, all this was after only the first test. The future valedictorian got into a lot of political turmoil by using his class presidency to lobby for us. And he successfully bailed us out. But his outspokenness cost him later, as we shall see. We tried to call out that charmer of a professor, but he was nowhere to be found, and by this time new professors were teaching their specialties in the course. Things only got worse. Even though the students woke up and started studying harder, the ensuing tests were unbelievably difficult. No one said a word to me about my previous predictions, but I did get some street cred. We finished the course with low averages, even with a substantial final curve. I finished with an 83, and that was the second highest grade in the class. It would have been nice to pillory that "certain" prof and make him eat those Levo and Dextro simple sugars until he became sick. By the way, he was the one prof at my interview that almost scuttled me, insulting my undergrad college, my acumen and me. I still got in; I still didn't like him.

19

I'm a Pigg

Freshman Histology was extremely stultifying; one of the hardest courses offered in dental school. You had to learn all about cells and be able to observe and identify them microscopically. Some lucky students had previously taken this course in undergrad; the rest of us just suffered. One day in Histo lab the stout Dr. Hogg was busy lecturing in her slow, deliberate and unyielding way when suddenly something humorous came over me. The atmosphere in there was dead quiet and very intense as I leaned over to a classmate and whispered, "You know, she has a sister named Ima." My friend burst out with loud guffaws that wouldn't stop and turned red-faced as well. Everyone froze and stared at him. What the hell was his problem? Did he really want to get killed by her? Professor Hogg stopped mid-sentence, sighed deeply, gave him a staredown and continued. Nothing happened. Boy, was he mad at me. We did make up later with profuse apologies on my part. In my defense, I didn't think that cornball joke was *that* funny. These serious city folk sometimes found levity in the most inane and juvenile discourses. It was unpredictable. However, I never heard him laugh in school again!

20

Dentists Versus Basic Scientists

Boy, what an epic battle this always was, or so I was told
by upperclassmen. The first two years of dental school had
its share of dental courses, taught largely by full and part-
time faculty, who were dentists. The rest of the courses, the
basic sciences such as biochemistry, histology, pharmacology,
physiology, oral cancer, anatomy, etc., etc., were taught
by Ph.D. professors employed by the college to teach and
conduct research. For some of them, teaching us bottom
feeders was beneath them, while others did a decent job. As
students, we naturally gravitated toward the "real doctors"
whom we would be like some day. The basic scientist Ph.D.'s
were foreign bodies to us and, in fact, a lot of them were
foreigners and difficult to understand. And most of them
didn't like us much either. There was always this undercurrent
of envy, or at least the perception of one. The lowliest full-
time dentist-educator made more money than the longest
tenured Ph.D. professor. Everyone knew it and kind of never
spoke of it in school. Anyhow, when it came to educating and

grading helpless students, we really got the shaft from the Ph.D.'s. They knew we only put up with their courses because we had to. They also keenly recognized our half-hearted efforts in their classes and labs. After all, we were going to be dentists, not scientists, and make big bucks someday. This kind of attitude was voiced on more than one occasion by fellow students during times of stress, frustration or simple arrogance. Not a good thing to say as a freshman. A little comeuppance was always in store for us if we bent scholarly rules in the least. It was a dicey game we played in order to learn from both types of doctors at our dental school, and to graduate without offending either too much.

21

Learnin' On Each Other?

How do you think we learned about those nasty-tasting and messy dental materials? That's right– we were forced to practice on each other, especially during first year. It was brutal, and all our efforts were harshly graded, to our chagrin. We were told not to eat before certain lab sessions. Barf buckets were strategically placed as ignorant students began shoving, placing and squirting waxes, sour pastes, vile solutions, and gooey impression materials in each others mouths. Not a pretty sight. Well, you couldn't let us loose on patients before we at least had a rudimentary knowledge of the stuff we would later use on them. It was a necessary evil. It was also surprising how few of us actually became sick; although some became quite ill from the poor grades they received! We choked but learned quickly and for the most part kept those barf containers empty. I went through a few ties, however.

22

First Cleanings

During the middle of first year, we were "clinically" introduced to dental hygiene by pairing off in the large periodontal laboratory and, under vigilant tutelage, "cleaned" each others teeth. Love taps at first, then stronger and deliberate strokes. No dental chairs, no overhead lights, no spittoons. You can imagine what kind of job we did– crappy! However, better us getting bloody and torn up gums than private paying patients. And, so we learned, and got graded for our efforts. Slowly but surely our dexterity improved, our grades rose, and the German-made, razor-sharp, metal instruments no longer felt foreign. By the end of first year, we set upon the populace, the one that was willing to let dental school *schlubs* work on it for a reduced fee. *Caveat emptor.* Hey, I think they got a good deal, maybe.

23

11 p.m. Hello

Communicating with a beloved partner and future spouse is not an easy task when cohabiting; it is plain daunting when living over four hours apart! Such was my situation upon embarking for dental school after successfully graduating from pharmacy college. I reluctantly left my fiancée's behind; behind to finish her pharmacy degree and then to eventually join me in married life. However, we had to get through two years of an unanticipated long distance engagement first. Skype, Instagram, Facebook were not invented yet, cellphones either. Even the "computer" at the time was rudimentary, at best. Email? What was that? The much maligned and scoffed at rotary telephone was our lifeline to each other back then; complete with a bulky hand held receiver and curly extension cord. And it was plugged into a land line, in the wall! Many phone plans of that era had a feature where calls after 11 p.m. were free, even on weekends. So, a whole town, a whole populous ended up phoning home at once, starting at that magical hour. People lined up at public pay phones in droves;

arguments and fights broke out. It was a crazy time; all that, just to talk to another human "for free." As relatively poor college students, this 11 p.m. perk was our life for a while. We only saw one another approximately once monthly, so the telephone was crucial to our relationship. Suffice it to say that whoever got to the phone first was golden. Normally amicable friends and roommates would often tussle and grapple with each other to get first dibs on that damn phone! The losers angrily glared at the early bird winners, paced the floor, pointed at the clocks, etc. Everyone wanted a turn as quickly as possible because it was late. No one wanted to stay up any later than necessary. My fiancée and I made it and eventually married anyway. Today's generational propensities for instant gratification and available technological marvels were unknown to us back in the day. Can you imagine telling a modern millennial that she/he had to wait until 11 p.m. to sext? It would be blasphemous, but funny!

24

Pasta, Pasta, Pasta

What does a relatively poor dental student eat in an expensive town? Well, for the first two years I dined on spaghetti, meatless sauce with an occasional hot dog thrown in. (Our dental school cafeteria was only open for lunch and was pricey.) It was almost a ritual with me. Two slices of pizza for lunch, angel hair noodles and spaghetti sauce for dinner, followed by a small cup of Taster's Choice decaf coffee. Then I hit the books hard until 11 o'clock, when I phoned my fiancée (calls were free after 11pm if you had our plan back then). Then, bedtime. The only variation of this routine was the choice of sauce: Prego, Aunt Millie's, Sano's, Ragu, etc. The sauce wars were all the rage in the early '80s. Which one was better? I ate them all, and loved them all. However, Prego was my favorite. Let me tell you, those first two years may have seemed austere by today's standards, and they were. And, it is also true that I lost about 20 lbs. But, I felt great, had energy and was arguably in the best mental state of my life. All I had to think about was dentistry, my fiancée and pasta sauce. Subtract the suffocating and manufactured stress of dental school and I would have returned to those days in a second.

25

Pizza, Again?

Upstate it's called pizza; in other parts of the country it's sometimes called a pie. It sounds more delicious if called a pie! Getting a lunchtime bite to eat between classes is great fun in a large town, if you can afford it! A spontaneous lunch time endeavor was often lost on us poor and dowdy students. We were not yet loaded professionals. We didn't dress the part or act it, either. The frivolous and finicky lot that could partake in costly culinary finery already had a TV show, called: Sex in the City. Anyway, my miniscule budget gave way to a daily routine. I frequented a very small hole-in-the-wall Italian pizzeria named, "Italian Pizzeria." It was across the street from the dental school and quite convenient to get to. I quickly became a stalwart and pushy persona as I made my daily sojourn into this busy and eclectic eatery. No one was going to cut in line ahead of me or get my piece of the action! Only Italian was spoken behind the counter by the two harried brother-owners as they rushed around filling orders and cashing out customers. The pies were huge, the slices thick. You couldn't complain about the size. The place reeked of garlic and oregano, just as it should have. Very authentic. Nick and Tony were stout, short, dark-haired no-nonsense men with sour expressions on their faces. You stood in line, you pointed at the slice you wanted, paid, and left. Very simple. They also had Sicilian, but nearly everyone chose the thin slices. And, very few toppings were ever ordered. Two hefty slices for $1.50 would fill me up until dinnertime. The dough was excellent, the sauce sublime. I was a pizza connoisseur (as were most students back then) and this dive was the best! We all went back to our respective afternoon clinics, slightly thirsty, and slightly stinky– like garlic and spice cologne. Our breath stank; thank goodness for the recent advent of mandatory gloves and masks! I survived until supper, which was usually another blast of cheap angel hair pasta (my favorite) with Prego spaghetti sauce. Not Sano's, Ragu or Aunt Millie's, but Prego. I liked what I liked!

26

Morning Nap

Very few of my fellow students realized just how much and intensely I studied. During the first two years (while engaged and not married), every evening, night and most weekends were consumed by hitting the books. Part paranoia, part perfectionism, and part fear all fueled my pursuit of staying in school and graduating. Interestingly, I never had this same zeal for learning as a pharmacy student. It's possible that dentistry was my true calling, or was it? Of course I had a freshman dental school roommate that literally carried a worn out pillow with him in order to study and sleep in libraries, in all-night cafes, on street corners, etc. He did become the valedictorian, but that's another story. I was never that extreme. I did need to sleep after staying up late nightly with my big nose in a big textbook. So, what better time to get refreshed than during the mostly wasteful part of every school day: the morning lectures. A large, dimly lit, warm auditorium with comfy velour seats and no coffee. Sleepy-time! As I settled into my favorite chair in the back row, behind a wide pillar, and slowly put my coat hood over my head, I would always notice my good friend next to me getting ready to take notes. Good for him. Once in a while, as the soporific lecture would drag on, I would temporarily rouse if something "important" was uttered or shown, but not often. As the years wore on, most of my classmates and professors accepted my eccentric behavior and motto: "Sit as far away from the lectern as possible so as not to pick up any bullshit from the professors." This was not entirely true, however. All lectures were tape-recorded and printed out, a bona fide transcript service started by a fellow classmate. We paid him a small fee and he did this for our class in all subjects. The administration did not object but resented some of the ensuing absenteeism. I was always present, but basically comatose. I ended up reluctantly reading the professors' bullshit via printed paper. However, as I suspected early on, most lecture material was hastily put together, faulty, incomplete or conflicting. *Hello* textbooks and old exams. I knew a few students that never cracked open a textbook, relying only on their hand-written notes and the transcripts. I wonder what they actually learned. My good friend W. took copious notes in class and went through many pens. I finished high up in the class, was never sleep deprived, and had ink to spare at graduation. I'm not being self-congratulatory, just honest.

27

Bogus Bookstore

It was bad enough being forced to purchase expensive dental instruments and sundries during freshman year, but then we had to continue the buying process to resupply our constantly dwindling cache. Just like in private practice, on our nickle, mind you! The logic was that much of this initial investment would be used to start our private practices upon graduation. Well, yes and no. Only the drills and non-disposable items held up. Waxes, liquids, acrylics, etc., were quickly used up. Sure, the various clinics had meager supplies, but those were only to be used after our personal "bought" supplies were exhausted. We were all watched very carefully by staff members. You couldn't go to a clinic supply desk without prior approval from a professor. The dental bookstore, however, was a smorgasbord of dental armamentarium– it had everything from plastic teeth to bib clips. And, the prices were outrageous. Yes, you had to pay through the teeth to continue learnin.' Cash only, no credit cards. Basically, it functioned as a mini cash cow for the school. As if a dental education wasn't costly enough! This was the convenient 7-11 to go to. We had no choice, and we went in droves, all the time, all hours of the day. The frugal and meticulous students saved money, others, not so much. The store employees were bonded sales people and not hired students. There was no favoritism or freebies. I swear, some lackadaisical students laid out mega bucks in this store. But, most of those saps were wealthy; what's a few drill bits between friends? My austere spending habits carried on after dental school and helped keep my overhead low in private practice. With some of my other fellow graduates, probably not so much.

28

Why Are You Here?

Why were any of us in dental school? Especially in the early '80s, with AIDS running rampant across susceptible communities and a mini-recession at hand. Times were tough, but any generation can say that in hindsight. At the time, we were all immersed in Dentistry 101, and blinkered to the outside world. Sure, we read and saw the daily news, but we were basically isolated and privileged professionals with loads of optimism. Things were going to get better, honest. New patients treated at our school had the potential of AIDS infection and that didn't scare us. Ronald Reagan stumbled out of the gate after beating Jimmy Carter and that didn't frighten us either. We were basically fearless. I believe most of us were there for the right reasons; you know, for duty and humanity (Three Stooges quote). However, you just knew that some were in it for money and glory, but what else is new? But, a few female students in my class and in other years were there for another reason– boredom. What? Not to pigeon-hole, but most of these ladies resembled one another.

All had stellar undergraduate grades from swanky "finishing colleges," decent DAT scores, and wore immaculate, expensive and stylish clothing. And some were actually cute, not good looking but cute. I remember asking one by chance why she was in dental school because she really exuded incompetence for this whole tooth business. She bluntly told me that her husband was a multimillionaire franchise owner of multiple McDonald's restaurants and she was a pampered, bored "JAP" with nothing to do all day. Was dental school the answer for chronic boredom, especially when also afflicted by millions of dollars? Evidently, yes. She also pointed out some of the other ladies in this unique "guild;" ones that I had already suspected of belonging. All had wealthy sugar daddy husbands that were very busy during the day. I don't know how seriously these women took dentistry or if they even practiced after graduation. I hope that someday I, too, can feel the wrath and despair of "affluenza" and feel their pain. I haven't felt it yet. And, I'm not bored either.

29

Double Gloving?

The AIDS crisis was in full bloom by the early '80s. It was first called HTLV III and not HIV/AIDS; it was the same thing. We freshmen dental students were justifiably alarmed and openly questioned our decision to enter a profession that dealt directly with this terminal disease. It was an epidemic, and transferable, although all the media and the CDC downplayed any contagious elements. I'm glad my parents and fiancée never realized just how bad things were. Then AIDS became politicized. We could not discriminate against any patient while knowing full well that many lied on the health history forms. "Just be careful" was a stupid axiom fed to us students. AIDS was now considered a disability as well as a deadly disease and infection. It was a tumultuous time for us. People were dying, it was constantly on the news, and there was no cure. Would we all eventually succumb and get sick? No one had any answers. The gay plague, gay cancer, good golly! The gay community was fighting hard to make HIV/AIDS legit and to not be ostracized from society. The rest of the populace didn't know what to do. Did I really sign up for this? Our school did the best it could in keeping us informed; it instituted mandatory universal protection policies. Gloves, masks, sharps containers, etc., were suddenly the norm. "Wet-fingered" dentists/instructors, used to working bare-handed, panicked. Wearing gloves was like wearing rubber condoms on your fingers, they exclaimed. Dexterity and touch would go out the window, or would it? We students didn't know any better; we started with gloves from day one. The dental professors protested half-heartedly. No one really wanted to die, after all. We all ended up getting used to wearing stuff on our faces and hands. Did all this get-up really help? No one knew for sure. It was the best we had at the time. Any patient who was bold enough to admit having HIV/AIDS got the special "sterile room," double gloves, gown, face shield and triple mask routine. Those were scary times. But we were too busy to realize the gravity of death from an "invisible" and seemingly ubiquitous virus. To the best of my knowledge, the only dental students and faculty that passed away due to HIV/AIDS were heavily involved in "alternate" lifestyles. No one got "it" from patients and, likewise, patients didn't get "it" from us. Well, here we are, thirty-five years hence and AIDS is still on the loose, in the news, and killing people. But we have learned so much more about it: Gays are not the only perpetrators, and heterosexuals in certain African countries are still dying from it. However, victims are less stigmatized and it is no longer a death sentence for healthy individuals. No antidote and a continuing scourge, yes, but manageable with the right drugs. However, those were rough times back then. I'm sure students and teachers violated many infectious disease safety protocols; nevertheless, none of us seemed to have become ill from this unintentional dereliction of duty. I guess HIV was harder to catch than we had thought. Who knew that the CDC would be right? Anyway, here's hoping future dental students and dentists have smoother sailing than we did.

30

Freshman Parties

"Lame" is the word I would best use to describe those ad hoc get-togethers of misfits seeking excitement. Always looking, but ultimately, not finding. You are what you are. However, it was still okay to attend those parties and at least poke fun at my fellow classmates. Sure, alcohol was present, sometimes in great quantities. And sure, people got silly, loud and obnoxious. It was all so juvenile and contrived. Parties in pharmacy college were honest expressions of joy, laughter and feelings. Many couples formed as a result of those mixers. Dental school parties seemed to be manufactured attempts at frivolity, but they were phony, like most of the students in attendance. Everyone wanted desperately to appear to be bon vivants; they just tried too hard. I wasn't fooled for a minute. These were gunners, cut-throats, and conniving two-faced back stabbers. They wouldn't have gotten this far in life if they weren't. I guess I was one of them, or was I? I remember telling my fiancée about these sorry soirees and I kept her entertained with outlandish and endless tales about all the "personalities" in my class. Well, she finally came to visit me about two months into my freshman year and, of course, I took her to a large party. Her stares of amazement and awe made me laugh out loud. She apologized profusely to me for ever doubting my stories. I had embellished and exaggerated nothing! She said she had never been introduced to so many geeks, dweebs, twerps, and misanthropes in her life. It felt good parading around my hottie blondie among the many toads that passed as women in my class. The men weren't much better. I'm not lying, I had a witness! We left the party that night and had an epiphany. Maybe it was time to invite dental students to my apartment and have a *real* party. My fiancée volunteered to come down again to help out. I'm sure my two roommates wouldn't mind. Now, this was a righteous and cool plan ('80s speak).

31

A Real Party

Back in the day, pharmacy college parties had been a riot. However, after attending a few lame freshman dental school parties, I realized something drastic had to be done. How about hosting a *real* party? I would be in charge of the planning, execution and horseplay; my roommates would lend a hand and give me some funds for the refreshments, eats and "party favors." We decided to have it on a Saturday night to accommodate all the Orthodox Jewish students wishing to attend (Friday night Shabbat– sorry). Also, we needed Friday night and Saturday morning to spruce up our place and get set up. Having already established myself in the first few months of freshman year as a bit of a fun-loving eccentric card, it took no time at all to circulate the news of this upcoming social. Most of the droll students seemed enthusiastic and many actually promised to attend. So far, so good. My lovely fiancée was going to come down that weekend and help me clean sweep the pad, buy the booze and Mary Jane, and get ready to rumble! Oh, did I mention that all my "buds" would be there: Sens, Panama Red, Hawaiian, Buddha Stick, Columbian Gold, and Thai Stick? Hash, no problem. Ask, and you would have received a bong hit, if necessary. Word kept spreading and even some cool professors asked about the address and time. This was going to be big, maybe huge. It was *HIGH* time someone held a proper mixer to Sens things up! Friday night and Saturday a.m. were also spent rearranging our one bedroom flat to have more room. My hottie blondie worked tirelessly mopping the floors, taking out garbage, washing, lifting, etc. Can't beat those upstate mountain girls– they're not allergic to hard work! My roommates helped with the money. Their wealthy and spoiled girlfriends did not help us in the least and were amazed at the effort put forth by my fiancée. They were both city "JAPS"; what did you expect? Perching and posturing in expensive adornments were their strong suits. It's funny how neither roommate ended up marrying either "princess." Our apartment– actually, the second one we lived in that first year– was a normal, third story, one bedroom, *illegal* sublet. It was close to the dental school and was owned by a sketchy and slimy recent dental school graduate who assured us things were on the up and up. When the building's super withheld our mail and accused us of being squatters, we got the hint. We ended up leaving after our freshman year, but not before that epic party. It was 6 p.m.; officially the festivities started at 8 p.m. Who was ringing that damn doorbell so early? We were still eating dinner and separating the seeds from the buds! Was it the asshole landlord coming by? No, it was Nathan T., the obnoxious and immature chubby Orthodox kid in our class. His yarmulke was flapping on his curly mop top as he bustled in and plopped a six-pack of very expensive brew on our table. He looked genuinely relieved that he was invited in and not instantly bodily removed. Hey, all of a sudden, he was okay in my book. Costly suds, I'm down! And, he acted okay all night. Other revelers remarked to me that he added great levity to the occasion. I guess he was still laughed at, and not with. Oh well, I don't think he knew. Slowly, more people filed in, professors, upper-classmen, men, women, LGBTQ peeps, etc. It became crowded in a hurry. Luckily, the hallway outside was spacious; our patrons took their hooch and hemp and *platzed* where they could find a space. None of the other tenants complained, some joined us. To be fair, we constantly had to turn down the stereo volume to be neighborly except when Manhattan Transfer was played. Then, my roommate— who absolutely loved them– would crank it up. People smoked, toked, joked, and drank. Most, if not all, had fun because of the positive atmosphere, music selection, and consumable/smokable goods available. No one got stupid, profs didn't hit on any freshmen chicks, and nothing got broken. The party ended at 1 a.m. and we just sat there, staring at each other and breathing sighs of relief. It was as if we had won a sporting event championship, or something. It was successful and satisfying. Months and years later, the *real* party was still talked about. Many students embellished the debauchery that never happened, and included my name in the tales. I didn't mind; all part of the dental school legacy and lore.

32

Walkman Woes

Before personal electronic devices, cell phones, I-pads, etc., there was the Walkman! This was the '80s, of course. It was a time when men were men and women dressed as men. Being taken seriously was in. Personal space was also getting smaller. The Walkman was a portable cassette recorder/ player with headphones for undisturbed music appreciation. It was brand new, exciting. You could now listen to your favorite records– literally take your Technics turntable with you on the street, as long as you had batteries and eight track cassettes available. CD discs later replaced the cassettes, and then technology really leapt forward. But for a short while, in the early '80s, the Walkman ruled! But not in dental school. A few "boundary pushing" dental students tried to use the Walkman in the long and tedious dental laboratories, especially during first and second year. Although it was true that the professors' instructions could not be heard by headphone ensconced students, it was also apparent that most professors relished the prospect of physically breaking the "new-fangled devices" in order to send a message. Overnight, the Walkman was officially outlawed by my dental school and that was it. No one violated the new rule, period. I wonder what happens in dental schools today? Do students covertly sext while cutting teeth in a mannequin head? Do professors watch and catch them, or are they themselves also busy sexting to really care? Drill, fill, and text in between; the new normal?

33

Do It Over

Ah, the popular mantra of my dental school. At least in the first year, when we were useless plebes just trying to gain a foothold in dentistry. However, this attitude and physical destruction of lab work continued until graduation! Nothing brought more glee to an instructor's face and extreme agida to a student than to hear the words "Do it over." Sometimes it was justified, sometimes not. It all depended on the mood of the instructor that day. Whims and moods are funny things. We thought that the "mental hazing culture" and the clobbering of dental work underfoot was just hearsay. It was not. I personally witnessed it, and it was awful. We had heard that other dental schools, like Stony Brook for instance, really took pride in their coddled, wimpy students and nurtured them along gently and kindly. Not so my school. It was known as the dental school of hard knocks and, boy, was that on the money! A typical episode would entail an enraged clinical instructor berating a lowly student in front of his peers and patient and then unceremoniously grabbing the "offensive" lab work (denture, crown, partial denture, etc.) and throwing it violently to the ground and then stomping on it to emphasize its shortcomings. Denture teeth and porcelain would go flying in all directions. The student would just stand there and take it (PTSD in later life?), the patient would be embarrassed, and the professor involved would joyfully exhalt in triumph– *Do it over*! You never knew when it would happen to you. Fortunately, I lasted all four years without any traumatic incidents, but I can't say the same for my close dental brethren. None of this was known to the public, unless you were a first-hand patient observer. And, nothing was ever reported to any higher authority. Those three words were permanently imprinted on all of our psyches forever. Did we become better dentists for it, or was legalized dental hazing at my school just part of the normal education and a right of passage? Sometimes you don't realize that it is abuse unless blatantly pointed out by an outsider. It was a tough-ass school and everyone knew it, yet no one dared to change things or file a complaint.

34

Cabs On Ice

There wasn't a funnier sight than witnessing the frustration and poor driving ability of taxi drivers when it snowed in town. Although the winters were generally mild, we did get some doozy storms, nonetheless. Coming from upstate N.Y., snowflakes didn't faze me. However, most of the cab drivers were foreign-born; many came from the Middle Eastern part of the world. I'm sure most had heard of the white stuff but never had to maneuver in it! Rear wheel drive cars, slick road conditions, and mindless hacks! That combo resulted in a kaleidoscope of yellow colors pointing in different directions and moving slowly. To see a free circus, I only had to look out my apartment window and gaze at the folly. They just didn't know how to drive in the stuff! What fun. Few fares were probably collected on snow *daze*; I bet most just went slip sliding away (Paul Simon).

35

The Instructor Debacle

We weren't just thrown into treating live patients. First, we had to practice on inanimate representations of the mouthparts (mainly teeth!) in large dental laboratories, sitting in rows behind huge, black marble-coated bench tops. Freshmen year introduced us to the various teeth, gums, dentures, partial dentures, etc. We had to learn everything from the ground up, even if it would never be useful as a "real" dentist some day. Hours and hours were spent drilling on plastic teeth, then real ones, as well as learning how to make dentures, and studying gum disease. These hands-on scenarios continued well into second year to sharpen our eye-hand coordination and learn about the oral cavity. Intense lecture portions supplemented the lab sessions and made dental school actually two schools in one. You were learning to be both a tradesman with good hands and a scientist with book smarts at the same time. It was a very difficult proposition, but necessary before students were let loose upon patients during the latter half of second year. My particular row in the removable prosthodontics lab (dentures) during first year was a mismatch of funky students: a former Chinese paratrooper, two Orthodox Jews, a former stripper, a former pharmacist (me), a former social worker, and a few "normal" but eclectic students thrown in. Our row instructor was a foreign-born, American-educated prosthodontist. She was a short-haired, short-statured and short-tempered bitch on stiletto heels. She was relatively young, attractive and seemed to have a lot to prove. We got off to a slow start that fall, being rather incompetent and all. I mean, we had never done this before. A few months in, however, it became apparent that all the other rows of students were progressing at a faster pace than we were and also having fun. We quickly became her "whipping boys." She berated us constantly for the full lab periods. Nothing was good enough for her, yet we were still behind the others. Finally, all ten of us row rats got together in private to discuss the ongoing misery and possible solutions. We just weren't learning from her. She sucked as a teacher. One of our row-mate's father, a prominent dentist and alumnus, offered to get involved and "straighten her out." We considered this option but opted for a written grievance petition to be submitted to the dept. head of the first and second year removable prosthodontics dept. This was a last gasp attempt to rectify the worsening situation prior to a mutiny, or at least a sit down strike! The dept. head was G3 (G cubed), a euphemism for GQ (the magazine) and the three first letters of his full name. He was a stunningly Hollywood-handsome, silver-haired prosthodontist, with a penchant for bedding willing freshmen ladies. The petition was written, copied and signed by all members of our row except me! Persuasion did not work on me; the petition was subsequently handed in, and we waited. During our next scheduled lab period, the "bitch on heels" was curiously absent and we just sat there leaderless, and waited for something to happen. We didn't have to wait long as the shit was about to hit the fan. G3 poked his head out from his corner office and started beckoning each of us in turn into his private den. After the first student exited with a glazed-over, frightened expression on his face, we knew we had stepped over the line, big time. But, what else could we have done? Multiple previous complaints fell on deaf ears and had only made the "bitch" angry, vindictive and more volatile. However, G3 had hired her and he was damn pissed off at us. How dare we challenge his authority? It was a deeply personal insult to him. My turn came and, as the door slammed behind me, G3 looked me straight in the eye and growled, "Mayputz, I didn't see your fuckin' name on this goddamn petition; why not?" I replied in an even voice, "I don't like to attach my name to any unproven cause. It's not worth it." He leaned back, paused, reflected on what I had just said, smiled, and uttered, "You're very smart, keep up the good work! Now, get the hell out of my office and send the next asshole in." The petulant and bitchy row instructor was indeed fired, a new one hired, and we finally caught up on our work. We had won, or did we? All nine of the petition signers received low grades in this lab and had "difficulty" passing other prosthodontics labs in ensuing years. But not me. Coincidence? Perhaps. G3 would always give me a wink and a smile whenever we crossed paths in the hallways. I think we both knew the truth.

36

Mr. Coney

You could always tell a freshman from an upper-classman by the stench of embalming fluid (mainly formaldehyde) emanating from her/his clothing during the first six months of school. Gross Anatomy lab was responsible for this malodorous scent among the living. Freshmen were virtually immersed in this stank from opening day, being initiated into the medical sciences with the Gross Anatomy lecture portion and laboratory. A huge and poorly ventilated room near the top floor of the dental school was filled to capacity with cadavers on tables. Unnerved, shaky students were obliged to break up into foursomes and select a body. Of course all we saw were vague human forms covered in tan-colored plastic bags. We bravely broke up into groups and stood next to "our body." My group included my Irish roommate and two Orthodox Jews, one of whom was female. What a fearsome foursome we made! So as not to cause mass fainting, the corpses were positioned face down. We were told to carefully peel back a bit of the plastic covering and expose about five square inches of back. Scalpels in hand, we began the agitated process of "getting the feel" of cutting flesh. Baby strokes at first; love taps at best. Maybe it was callousness or bravado, but those first tentative forays as "surgeons" rather quickly morphed into students eating their lunches while perched over their fully dissected cadaver bodies! After each lab period, we dutifully sprayed our "body" with embalming fluid and carefully wrapped it back up with the plastic sheets. Our "body" wasn't the ideal specimen for dissection; fatty with poorly defined organs, nerves, arteries, etc. Other cadavers that were lean provided a much better teaching environment. Oftentimes all four of us would step away from our specimen and learn from a neighboring one. Our body never received any student visitors. On Fridays, at least once a month, I had to cut out of the lab early to make the 4:30 Trailways bus to visit my fiancée. My two Orthodox lab partners also had to duck out due to Shabbat, leaving the Irish *goy* to cover for me. I was never reprimanded for leaving the lab early. Either the professors thought I was Orthodox and just kept forgetting my yarmulke or my roommate kept coming up with ingenious excuses. No one on the bus complained about my stinky countenance; however my lovely fiancée made me strip upon my arrival to her apartment, which was just fine by me! Gross Anatomy ended and no one had passed out. Thank you Mr. Ornell Coney for donating your body to science.

37

Cheating

Now, mind you, this is before the era of cell phones and today's technology. But, somehow, even in those prehistoric times, some tech-savvy students managed to participate in freshmen cribbing to beat the system. After all, these were the obnoxious go-getter students, the kind that did what it took to get ahead. The kind that looked through you instead of at you because they had better things to do than waste their time with you. School was to be conquered and Porsches to dream about. These certain "smart guys" looked and acted liked seasoned doctors after just a few days in school. Confident, articulate, and full of bravado. The bullshit artists! You know who I mean. Gross Anatomy lab practicals were difficult. Sometimes internal body parts all looked the same. They were not color-coded! The collusion of cheaters used some sophisticated wiring and mics (by '80s standards), all bought at Crazy Eddie stores. The smartest of the bunch would whisper the answers during the practical into the top of an innocuous looking pen and his cohorts would receive the messages via poorly concealed ear buds. Virtually foolproof! But not all professors were fools, as we found out. The scheme was exposed and the cheaters discretely expelled. I wonder if these former students "made it" in life? Are they selling ice to Eskimos and driving Porsches? I'd like to know.

38

Cash is King

I was behind J.T., in line at the Bursar's office payment window. It was time for second semester payment during my freshman year. I had a check in hand; J.T. had a brown paper bag in hand. Lunch? No way– he carefully opened it and slid wads of Benjamins underneath the bulletproof glass window to the Bursar's secretary! She seemed nonplussed, staring at him, unblinking. Thirteen grand in cash. Well, this might explain why he was still enrolled. You see he was a consummate weasel and bullshitter. He also put the *I* in inept. His older brother and father had been honor graduates of our school but J.T. was not cut from the same cloth. He had managed to bluff and buffalo instructors during the first semester and was obviously aiming to continue doing the same crap. We fellow students had no use for him and detested his bravado and bluster. He finally was called out on his very poor grades and lab performances by a lowly, insignificant secretary, of all people. Word spread quickly and he was summarily bounced from our fine institution. But wait, I found out after graduation that he was back in school again. What? Why? How? Evidently being a legacy helped, and cash was still king.

Take a break!

SOPHOMORE YEAR

39

Boy Bruce

I decided that second year would be different and better, as far as room and board went. I had successfully browbeat the dental school housing director into "finding" me space. His office and policies were a joke and everyone knew it. Out-of-state, upstate, and international students were often frozen out of the limited dorms while local "connected" students got in. No one knew how this system worked. I didn't get a spot my freshman year and expensive private accommodations just added to my stress. After berating the director for a few minutes over the phone during the summer before second year, he acquiesced and magically found room for me. If you don't ask, you don't get! The dorms were cheaper and close to the dental school. A win-win situation for me, or so I thought. But I was going to have a roommate. What could possibly go wrong? The super in the previous building I had lived in was elated to see me and my two roommates vacate the premises; we had been illegally subletting for a year and didn't know it. My parents and I successfully extricated my meager belongings from the flat I had shared, got them loaded up in a pull-behind trailer, and carted them to the dental dorm building, about twenty minutes away. Before we started unloading, my folks and I decided to first check out the pad. It was about two weeks before school commenced, so no one should have been there. We rode the elevator to the sixth floor, I took out the key but knocked on the door, just in case. To our surprise, out popped a Sean Hayes look-alike, who proceeded to give me a winsome smile and a limp-fish handshake. "Hi, my name is Bruce," he lisped. He was handsome, clean-cut, well-spoken, and somewhere over the rainbow. My mother remarked how well-mannered and groomed he was. My father was clueless. My first thoughts were that the housing director had gotten even with me for my hubris. Damn him! Bruce was going to be my roommate for the whole year! Could I take it? I wasn't sure. But it was too late. He was a senior, so we would only be living together for that one year. That was encouraging. Strangely, I had heard of him as a freshman but never paid much attention to that scuttlebutt. Maybe I should have. Jogging my memory bank, it seems that he was portrayed by other students as exceedingly smart, gifted and very flamboyant. Great, just great. Our beds in the large studio dorm room were a mere six feet apart; we would be sleeping in the same room! The tiny room had one closet, a small kitchen, a puny bathroom and Bruce. Good thing I was low maintenance because it could have gotten ugly fast. I was moved in, my folks departed in a happy mood, and I was left with Bruce. He was over the top in mannerisms, speech and lifestyle. It was then and there, within the first few weeks of my second year, that I started calling him Boy Bruce (after Boy George). He loved the nickname and started calling himself that. My friends in school couldn't help ribbing me about him with inferences and innuendos about his life and peccadilloes. I quashed all the rumors by ignoring them and sticking up for him. After all, he was neat, clean, considerate, etc. He was shaping up to be a decent roommate. Our living arrangement was simple: I studied all the time, mainly in the dental school library until 11 p.m. nightly; he spent most of his time out on the town until the wee hours of the morning. He frequented "manly" establishments where numerous sexual encounters on a nightly basis were the norm. He would prep and preen himself prior to these trysts, and that included marijuana. He would often nonchalantly leave a dime bag of dope on my desk and I would roll him some bones and keep one for myself. That was our deal. I was an expert roller and had many compliments from those that indulged with him. I often feigned jealousy at his nightly sojourns which made him laugh. He sarcastically and gleefully suggested that I accompany him on some of his nightly jaunts; I ruefully declined. Can all you heterosexual men just imagine walking into a straight bar filled with attractive women and within an hour having sex with many of them? And not coerced sex, and not sex for money, but sex for fun and pleasure. And, with no strings attached! Such was his personal life. Unfortunately, my lot was listening to and remembering his steamy stories against my will. I'll never forget them, damn it! And I'll never, *ever* forget two of his favorite sayings: "Lay down you hot tramp" and "If I could lick my own balls, I'd never go out." Dentally, he was revered by many students and faculty alike. He was the youngest dental student in his class and had great talent and aptitude for dentistry. Everyone knew it and basically cut him some slack when it came to his frequent outlandish and bawdy behavior. He was Madonna, Boy George and Tommy Tune, all rolled into one, without the pipes, however. So the year went by. I was studying; he was partying nonstop, and was getting ready to graduate and move on. Even so, he managed to win a coveted senior dental student table clinic award about the Oral Manifestations of Aids and garnered much national and international publicity and praise. Such was his genius. I can honestly say that for a year we lived peacefully and happily together. He loved my fiancée and vice versa. They would compare shoes and makeup whenever she visited me. And in turn I liked all his "friends," but out of courtesy to me none ever stayed over. He often remarked that I was the best roommate he ever had. I believed him. We had no arguments, no spats and I never judged him. After graduation, he went on to do a prestigious general dentistry program at a VA hospital and was subsequently named the youngest dental director of the Aids treatment section of a major city hospital. He deserved it and I was really proud of him. We met for the last time at a continuing education seminar at which he was the featured presenter. It was the last year of my prosthodontics residency and I wanted to hear him lecture. He was happy to reconnect with me, but appeared tired, gaunt and worn out. He succumbed to Aids a few years later. I miss him; he was a good man. Over the years, I have sadly lost more than a few former classmates to Aids. Unfortunately, the LGBTQXYZ community, although mainstream and trendy, is not disease-proof.

40

Future Plans

We were all going to be dentists, at least in the conventional sense. Many conversations during the difficult second year often turned to thoughts of fanciful outcomes. Maybe it was the stress, or low blood sugar. Nevertheless, many classmates had it all figured out. I didn't, but listened in amusement to the chorus of know-it-alls. Blah, blah, blah. A millionaire owner here, a Maserati owner there, etc. Same old, same old. However, a few students did evoke some provocative and interesting futures for themselves, often to the derision of my classmates. Some of those future careers involved mixing dentistry with certain "hobbies," such as: Israeli tank commander, Zulu tribal chieftain, kibbutz manager, part-time porn star, stripper, D.J., rabbi, and big game hunter. There were probably more that I didn't remember. Now, some of that ignorant and self-righteous crowd did become rich and famous, although not many, and only a few that actually predicted it. However, *all* of those off-the-wall hobbies mentioned by that weird minority became reality for them, down to the stripping, pole dancing, gyrating, full monty displaying, hot-pants wearing man we simply called "Z." Out of courtesy, he had always worn a G-string under his dental scrubs as a student, or at least that's what I heard!

41

Knockoff

It was a cold, rainy, miserable day in November, and my watch had stopped. I didn't have time or money to take it to a jewelry store to have the battery changed, etc. And my father, an amateur but brilliant horologist (watchmaker), could have easily repaired it had he lived closer to me. Unfortunately, I had to find another remedy for my nonworking timepiece. I was on the way to class, fending off raindrops with my umbrella, when I was suddenly approached by a sinister-looking, trench coat-wearing, tall, black gentleman. He must have noticed that I was missing a wristwatch. He didn't speak, just planted himself in front of me, blocking my path forward. I gave him that knowing glare of not being born yesterday. My eyes told him to either "bring it" or clear out. I wasn't in the mood for bullshit. He instantly opened his huge coat to reveal numerous watches hanging from the lining. It was no cliché; gray market sales and service were the norm in this town. And, he was offering these products in broad daylight, although he did nervously scan the streets for the fuzz. I knew it and didn't care. "How much," I asked. "One Benjamin," he replied. I didn't want to play around and haggle. So, I immediately low-balled him with a price of $35, take it or leave it. I lowered my shoulder like a good running back to outmaneuver him when he grabbed said shoulder and planted a "Rolex" in my hand. He parted with a $20 watch, I parted with $35. We parted company and he quickly vanished into the streets. So, that's how I procured a genuine Rolex knockoff. I still wear it to this day. If mugged, I will readily give it up to a foolish thief. Let *him* try to sell it. He might get thirty five bucks for it, or less!

42

Temple in Situ

I wasn't the only "character" in *shul*. Far from it. Come to think of it, there were many. Very few students just blended in. Each had some unique quirk or special talent. Our dental school rabbi was no exception. Yes, we had our own rabbi! Actually, he was the only authentic rabbi in the entire school during his four year tenure. I had to ask him why he was here? He rubbed his fingers together in the money sign gesture. Besides, his congregation was dwindling and basically floundering. His words, not mine. Here was a stuttering, diminutive, glasses-wearing, religious scholar with a gross dental ineptitude and possibly an even greater deficit as a man of God. But, no matter. By his second year he actively sought me out as a tutor for all those darned ology courses: pathology, physiology, pharmacology, etc. The trade-off was old tests. Many students possessed some old dental exams, he just happened to have tons more of them, and for every year! I never asked where he procured them from ("Don't ask, don't tell policy"). I helped him to study, the old tests helped me get high grades. Another benefit of our friendship (friends with benefits?) included being invited to the myriad of Jewish holiday services, right inside the school. Witnessing him blow the shofar (special ram's horn) while dressed in a white lab coat was indeed a sight to behold. It was ironic that many of the attending professors were the same ones giving him D's in their dental courses. No favoritism for God's favorite. It was always comical to enter one of these religious services and have all the Jews give me the once-over. What's *he* doing here? The rabbi would politely explain that I was his special invited guest. I would sit quietly, politely eat the blessed food offerings, and chit chat with the dean of the college, the vice-dean, multiple chairmen of departments, professor-types, and fellow students. Not one of them ever questioned my presence or beliefs. I was amused but at the same time respectful and grateful to be taken into the confidence of this cabal. Our lone rabbi graduated on time with the rest of his class. And, please, call him *Doctor.*

43

Friday Exodus

The religious Jews, primarily males living under the tight dome of a yarmulke, were officially allowed to leave the school before sunset on Fridays. As Shabbat started on Friday evening, this privilege was non-negotiable and a given at my dental school. It was often disconcerting sitting in bowed drudgery, working furiously in a mandatory dental laboratory, only to look up at 4:15 p.m. and see huge swaths of missing students. Sundown started at 4:30 p.m. in November. And where was our fearless professor? Was he missing in action as well? I thought only Orthodox Jews received dispensation to vacate and rush home to their dimmer switches and already switched-on-ovens. It seemed like a disproportionate amount of students turned Jewish on Friday afternoons to get out early. There was no surveillance, accountability or testing of piety. I had an emergency yarmulke in my locker just in case of trouble, but I never used it. Maybe I should have. We remaining diehard gentiles would sometimes make callous remarks about the absenteeism; perhaps we were just jealous.

44

The Italian Contingent

It seems that I have been mentioning and alluding to a large Jewish presence at my alma mater. Well, it was true. However, there was also a large block of Italian-American students and professors. They comprised at least 30 percent of the class. Now, my school was very ethnic in nationalities and religions. No one was a mere American mutt, well, maybe one or two per class. The majority of the student body very proudly sported their overseas bloodlines. The Jewish fraternity had its members, as did the Italian fraternity. And the group members tended to hang out with each other as well. I was used to regular American kids; I was usually the oddball "foreigner." Not so in dental school. Everyone was proud of her/his heritage and wore it on their sleeves, so to speak. I got along fine with the Italian crowd; they thought I was Catholic. I got along fine with the Jews, after I told many that I was Orthodox. Well, Orthodox Estonian, that is.

45

Son of Odin

He was known by reputation as the oddball professor, a part-time Fixed Prosthodontics row instructor who actually cared and taught students something. Fixed Prosthodontics (crowns, bridgework, implants) was a very laborious desk top laboratory course during the second year. It was grueling to learn the manual nuances of drilling shapes and forms and also difficult to teach. He was an "unreal" character, complete with a Norwegian accent frequently laced with vulgar profanities. And, he didn't care who he good-naturedly insulted; it was all in good fun. At least it was for him. We were all lucky enough to have him as a prosthetics row instructor during that second year because our row was the same collection of inane dunces as in the previous year. Alphabetical order in a large class is a bitch. I was stuck with these row-mates for the duration. And he had his work cut out for himself trying to train us up to be dentist types. He had a large and successful general practice in town and really didn't need the aggravation of teaching us boneheads. But he did, nonetheless. He was very gifted as a dentist with an outsize personality to match, and he started our dental learning from day one. No nonsense but with a wicked sense of humor; it was a delight to interact with him. His "true" stories of moose hunting in Norway, eel fishing in the fjords of Sweden, and working for the CIA during WWII were legendary. He still had a full carry pistol permit which he showed us, and made allegations that he was packing all the time. No one wanted to cross him! But he was beloved by all, students and other instructors alike. We learned *not* to cut a tooth that looked like a "cat's dick," learned to make temporary crowns that fit tightly, like a "rubber," learned that hard work and perseverance paid off, and learned that smoking cigarettes during the lab period was for row instructors only. What a teacher, what a personality! I have never met anyone like him since. He was an original. I graduated without thanking him and for that I am truly sorry. He put the b in bizarre, but without him and his personal encouragement, I wouldn't have become a prosthodontist. I miss him.

46

Cockroach Delight

My future father-in-law, Joe, was coming to town for a numismatic conference (coin show) and wanted to stay somewhere cheap. How about my dental dorm room? My roommate would be out of town that weekend; it was a no-brainer. Joe and I had hit it off famously the very first time we met, about four years prior. It would be no problem hosting him. In fact, it would be a pleasure. The weekend started out on Friday with him buying me dinner at a very swanky rib place. After two double Manhattans each, we weren't feeling any pain, or anything, for that matter. The ribs were fantastic as was the onion loaf appetizer, a house specialty. Always the wine connoisseur, Joe ordered us a particular red wine to go with dinner. I didn't complain. The cab ride to the dorm building was laughter-filled, with two drunk gentlemen in the back seat. Of course, we took a Checker cab. He loved it, just like in the movies. (They were slowly phased out in the '80s as a car company.) We stumbled into the elevator of my building and finally fell into my apartment. It had been an exhausting day for both of us and just being able to collapse with no further responsibilities was a relief. He had the show the next day and I had studying to do. But tonight, we were going to live it up. Too bad we were already tired and ready for bed at 9 p.m.! I cracked a few Moosehead lagers to get things started. There was Mets baseball on my small black and white TV, and I had corn chips. Let's get this party started! Both of us started to nod off almost immediately; baseball can be a soporific game. However, we both managed to get a second wind after indulging in a Sens blunt. The talking and laughter started back up and we had some lively and profound conversations, if only I could remember them. Maybe it was the Moosehead/Sens combo? Anyway, time for bed. He would sleep in my roommate's bed with new sheets. Simple. Brushing, flossing, urinating, and then– lights out. At around midnight, I heard a loud yell come from the kitchen area. I turned on the lights to find Joe standing there in his boxers transfixed, like he saw an alien or something. He asked me if the room was spinning. And, was the paint spotted in the kitchen? It was just the roaches, hundreds swarming the kitchen in their nightly foraging ritual. Being drunk and high made it seen unreal or surreal, whichever. Joe had gotten up to get a glass of water and didn't expect the overwhelming welcoming committee in the kitchen, and I had not forewarned him. We had a good laugh and went back to bed. The building's super knew every apartment was infested, but we were lowly dental students, and only here for a short time. So it really didn't matter. My future father-in-law was a cool dude. He had taken it all in stride and actually admitted years later to having had a good time with me. I ended up marrying his eldest daughter and we also lived in that same apartment for a few weeks after our wedding, at the end of my second year. Like her father, my new bride was cool, and the cockroaches didn't bother her one bit. Maybe that's a good way to test out a prospective mate. Let her sleep with the roaches for a night and see if she still talks to you the next morning. We're still married.

47

Drillin' and Fillin'

This was the early '80s and silver amalgam (yes, the one with elemental mercury in it) still dominated operative dentistry as the popular tooth filling material of choice. Durable though unsightly, it was technically easy to manipulate and condense. It was, and still is in many practices, a tried and true restorative substance for filling cavities. An oldie but goodie. Although the "white" fillings (plastic composite—basically a soft resin conglomerate with fine filler particles for strength, hardened by a blue wavelength curing light) are now state of the art and done by most dental offices, silver amalgam is still around. They let us loose on real live patients during the latter half of second year, after demonstrating proficiency by correctly drilling and filling first plastic, and then real extracted teeth, on a bench top in a laboratory setting. That lab training took a while; some students progressed to patients faster than others. All of first year and part of second year were consumed by intense lab sessions, with billowing clouds of tooth dust rising up from around bespeckled dental initiates, drilling away the faux decay. Then came plugging, carving, shaping and polishing the silver. Of course a real patient had things like saliva, nerves, a tongue, head, lips, etc. Things that got in the way. Things that you had to learn to navigate around. Anesthesia? Shit, forgot about that! Well, the professors started us off easy. They screened the patients for easy cavities to make sure we newbies could handle things. Nothing too deep; no root canals! At least, not yet. And *they* gave the anesthesia before letting us rip. I remember my first operative patient, an elderly, soft spoken black gentleman who came to our school and clinic to save a buck. He was genial and a delight to interact with. After reviewing his operative needs, a professor got him numb and I started, just like that. The suction apparatus was faulty, there were no assistants to help out, his tongue was constantly in the way, the lighting was poor, etc. But, after three sweaty hours I managed to place a large silver filling. I took off my latex gloves, wiped my brow and took off my face mask. The patient was grinning with pride for my sake. After waiting in line for an instructor, the work I did was scrutinized and graded. I received an honors grade. A good start. There was a long learning curve ahead for me and my peers when you figure that a filling of that size now takes me approximately 15 minutes start to finish. Back then, just managing to get one filling done per three hour clinic session was enviable. That's how we learned: slowly, carefully, deliberately. Excavating decay and placing restorative agents were dentistry's bread and butter back then, and still are today. Dental materials have changed dramatically over the decades but teeth haven't; most dentists are microsurgeons/microengineers of the oral hard tissues (teeth) and continue to drill and fill!

48

Blow Jobs Forbidden

We were second year dental students and he should have known better; obviously he did not. Even though sterility protocols were absent in the laboratory setting, it was still impressed upon us that certain things were taboo, such as blowing on a denture set-up to clean off wax shavings, etc. We were basically whittling and the natural inclination was to blow off the extraneous dribs and drabs, using your breath. Well, that was a big no-no. The logic was that this unacceptable behavior would translate into a later manifestation of blowing on a real denture and then inserting it into a live patient's mouth– gross! This one student was repeatedly warned but he could not stop from doing it. Although humiliated and apologetic, he was nonetheless ejected from the denture lab multiple times like an unruly baseball manager. He was a good guy, though. He didn't do it on purpose, he just couldn't help himself. He did make it to the end and graduated with the rest of us. Maybe keeping his face mask on in front of patients finally cut short that blowing habit of his? Let's hope!

49

The Three P's

I wished it was porn, porn and porn. But, alas, it stood for pathology, pharmacology and physiology, a bad trilogy, or should I say tragedy, for most dental students. We were warned about them and sure enough they hammered us during second year. I had taken physiology and pharmacology in pharmacy college so at least I could concentrate more on pathology. But even so, pharmo and physio turned out to be bears, and although I received A's, they were not easily earned. Most students received substantially poorer grades than I did, even with the curves. Pathology was difficult. It was taught by a consortium of non-dental professors and really tested our cranial cortex. Labs included gross dissections of diseased organs and tons of microscopic slides to study and memorize. The lab practicals were sobbing sessions for the weak minded or unprepared. The actual exams were long, taxing affairs that often left students mentally and physically altered for days afterward. We were going to be dentists, not physicians. What the hell? If you ask most general dentists in private practice about physiology, they will tell you they know where the mouth and tongue are, and how they work. If you inquire about pathology, they will tell you about what appears abnormal and sending a patient to an oral surgeon for a biopsy. And, pharmaceutically speaking, Amoxicillin and Lortab/Vicodin are basically the go-to drugs. All that study, all those all-nighters, all that coffee. What a waste?

50

Dental Darts

Time was at a premium in dental school. After studying, eating, sleeping, attending classes and labs, there was precious little of it left over for personal unwinding. Laundry, food shopping and worrying also took up a large chunk of it. That's why our weekly dart games during second year were so eagerly anticipated and so much fun. Fun, what's that? It was ironic that we worked with sharp syringes all day long, similar to darts. My second year dental cohorts and I descended on G.'s dorm room apartment on Thursday evenings and started shooting. He had a sweet setup, with a "professional grade" Winmau bristle board, proper lighting, and metal "English" darts. I brought my own darts (Voks Destroyer EL-C no bounce-out darts, with hot pink flights, weighing 24 grams each). I had been a bit of a player in undergrad and knew my way around the numbered circle either drunk, sober, or with my eyes closed. Here, in dental school, I quickly showed those pikers how to stand and deliver triples! I wish we had played for money. I still mentally relish those evenings which were wistfully spent throwing, laughing, and popping more than a few cold ones. I distinctly remember Pabst and Moosehead Lager as being our staple brews. After I left the dorms the following year, our "league" fell apart, but it was great while it lasted. I can still aim and shoot; occasionally my grown offspring and I go at it in my basement when they come to visit. Of course, my setup is "professional grade," I use the same darts, and it's still fun!

51

Trust and Confidence?

The worst patient response I ever received as a dental student occurred during second year. It was: "God-fucking damn it doc, it didn't hurt till you drilled it. Now I might need a root canal? That's horseshit!" He was a rather burly return customer and not in the mood for excuses or levity. Variations of his sentiment have occasionally occurred throughout my dental career and it still hurts each time I hear it. We were particularly vulnerable as dental students because we had no quick recourse for a "troublesome" patient. We were just measly students, trying to build confidence in our dental abilities and trust with our school patients. It was an awful feeling when dentistry went awry. What made it worse was the realization that often the patient or the tooth was actually at fault: the cavity was deep and close to the nerve to begin with, the patient expected heroic dentistry to "fix" a badly damaged tooth, etc. Unrealistic expectations on the patients' part often ruined the day. Conversely, too much patient education, vacillation and timidity on the student's part often did not instill confidence in the patient, either. It was often a soul-sucking and painful standoff for both parties. What a depressing profession to be in, huh? Patients didn't know teeth and dental students were just learning about them. How could a student develop faith in her/his abilities when constantly being dashed against the rocks of dental biology and patient recalcitrance? How did I handle that long-ago patient who accused me of "ruining" his tooth? Well, patient education, sincere apologies, and possibly waving his fee helped assuage his anger, somewhat. Ultimately, his forceful dismissal from the clinic by a stooped, elderly dental instructor finally sealed the deal. This old-timer had obviously witnessed our altercation and intervened. He firmly told the patient that the filling I had placed was fine, the bite was right on, the x-ray looked normal, and to be patient for a few weeks time. He then unceremoniously and physically escorted the bewildered patient out of the clinic in a bum's rush, and out of my hair (when I used to have some)! The dentist returned with a spring in his step, winked at me and said, "That's nothin'. Wait till you practice for a few decades." He was right, of course. I never saw that dentist in the clinic again after the incident, or that patient, for that matter! And, no one knew that dentist's name when I asked questions about him. Regardless, he saved me and I thank him. Who knew patient management could be that easy?

52

Catcalls

It was great sitting undisturbed in the back of the large and dimly lit main auditorium during all those tranquilizing second and third year morning lectures. I could doze unimpeded, look around at my nervous fellow classmates and even shout out things periodically to break up the tension. What? That's right, someone had to interject some much needed and well-timed levity into those monotonous, droning orations. Hey, it was appreciated by the class because people laughed, and laughed hard! That was the pay-off to my farcical remarks. So, I sporadically continued the entertainment. Why not? I believe the professors knew that I was the responsible culprit and perpetrator who often stymied their speeches. I also believe that my extremely high GPA and dental skills probably saved me from expulsion or at least any disciplinary action. Maybe "they" had senses of humor too and actually laughed along quietly during my "funny" outbursts? Possibly. I do know that no one in authority ever said a word to me, ever. Green light, baby! The head of the oral surgery department sometimes made a magnanimous entrance to a lecture to spew forth his "great" knowledge onto us neophytes. What an honor, what a man, what a fucking joke! I personally witnessed his hand-shaking extractions. Not a pretty sight. But he was revered and idolized at my school. He did have a gift for gab, however, and always talked his way out of obvious malpractice situations on the floor, often while demonstrating "easy" extractions to us, on already anesthetized patients. A clever tongue is sometimes better than a clever hand? His lectures were disjointed, opinionated, and basically a waste of our time. What a golden opportunity for me to get in some playful jabs. His topic that morning was about an infectious connection that sometimes occurred after a botched extraction (he should know) between the nasal cavities at the base of the nose (antral) and the oral cavity (oro). He repeatedly referred to this particular malady as an oro-antral fistula, although, it sounded like he was saying "oriental" and not oro-antral. Students looked around at each other uneasily and were confused. Was this a new kind of lesion, an "oriental" kind? Did it affect only Oriental people? What was he talking about? I was also thrown off. So, I started to mock him. Every time he uttered the word oro-antral I yelled out oriental. This went on for a few minutes, with students rolling their eyes and chuckling warmly. He kept stopping and finally said, "Is there an echo in here?" He wasn't laughing, just getting more and more sweaty and agitated by the minute. A very serious-looking, female, Asian-American "brown-nose" from the front row eventually walked up on stage and whispered to him that she didn't appreciate being disrespected and her culture ridiculed (at least that's what she told us later). He stood frozen and motionless, then proceeded to stalk off the stage to catcalls and laughter. Mission accomplished, as George Bush once said! We had about five minutes left in the class and most of the students turned around and saluted me in gratitude. I smiled warmly in return. The "Instigator" had won, at least round one. Unfortunately, we did get to hear "his majesty" again and again for the rest of the course. I didn't press my luck with any more forays into the humor realm, however. I think he knew I was responsible for his previous debacle and always gave me that pissed off glare after each one of his ensuing lectures. Oh well, it had all been in good fun. I'm just glad the N-word was never involved by accident. The Reverands Al and Jesse would have had a field day with that one!

53

Spare Time?

H*a, ha, ha.* Spare time in dental school? What a joke. We had so little of it. School was rough and the daily pounding by the professors reinforced that notion. We were like little nails being driven home by jackhammers. Hammertime! Anxiety alone seemed to eat up a lot of time. However, let's be honest. I wanted to excel and was a bit of a worrywart. My fiancée constantly reminded me that it was all my doing! Other students did not have their foot on the accelerator like I did and probably had a more balanced dental school experience. Of course my upcoming wedding had the potential to change everything. Perhaps even for the better? At least that's what I told myself. Hopefully I would be able to carve out some time again, for my wife's sake. Perhaps marriage would force me to better prioritize my life. And, hopefully my telomeres would stop shrinking as much. Spare time? Where did it go? I missed it through bachelorhood and marriage, and still do now. I guess I didn't change all that much after all, darn it!

54

Nuptials vs. the Pharmacology Final

The pharmacology final and my wedding weekend were on a collision course. I adamantly implored the head professor, whose book we used, to excuse me and give me a different date for the test; maybe even a harder exam if she felt like punishing me. "You're a pharmacist, why are you worried? You should ace this test," she barked sarcastically. Point taken. On the other hand, it was my wedding, damn it! So what, the pharmacology final was *obviously* more important. I always suspected that my dental-school-of-hard-knocks was "cold," and this episode confirmed it. No breaks given and none taken. I got hitched to my lovely fiancée on schedule that Saturday in June, did not review anything pharmacological over the weekend, and sat for the test on Monday morning. Our honeymoon had been wisely postponed until August, when school was out. I received the second highest grade on the final and finished the course with the highest average. I suppose that professor's faith in me had been justified after all. Although I could easily have taken a make-up final and avoided the unnecessary extra angst. However, this was PU College of Dentistry, where student suffering was a noble aspiration. I'm still mad at that bitch!

Take a break!

JUNIOR YEAR

55

The Marriage Paradigm

After being engaged at long distance for two years, we were finally united, and got married, too! My wife had graduated, eventually passed the pharmacy boards, and joined me as a legitimate spouse in my tiny dental dorm room. My previous dental roommate, Boy Bruce, had graduated and moved out. Nobody in the dorms said anything about my wife living there, although even the super knew she didn't belong. All was cool. No rat finks to rat us out. I was grateful for the many friendships I had forged. We were only there for a few weeks until the school year ended, then left for a three week belated honeymoon to Florida in my old college car. It was a beat up 1970 Plymouth Valiant that my father had valiantly refurbished, just in time for our trip. We followed up that wonderful trek with new digs in the LGBTQ part of town, and started living as a newly wedded couple. My wife quickly found employment as a pharmacist at a major drugstore chain and started the full-time *schlep*. The biggest challenges for me now were: increase in weight, decrease in studying time, decrease in my GPA, increase in overall worry, and monetary anxiety. Welcome to the world of marriage! Fortunately, third year was slightly less tortuous than the previous two years, so I wasn't overly concerned. Nevertheless, the pressures of marriage sometimes butted heads with the pressures of dental school. It was inevitable. I also didn't realize how many dental students in my class had tied the knot. How did they manage to do it all; some even had kids! However, to be honest, things could have been much, much worse for me. I was never dragged to go shopping, dancing or clubbing. My wife knew the importance of my dental education and was uncomplaining, supportive and accommodating. I got lucky marrying a beautiful, tough, low-maintenance, upstate mountain girl. We survived and thrived. My GPA suffered a bit, and my BMI ballooned slightly due to consuming more than pasta. So what? Life marched on and we had gone to the next level, having successfully navigated a few bumps in the dental/nuptials road along the way. There would be many more bumps to negotiate in the future. By the way, we're still married, to each other!

56

We're All Gay

Before my third year, my lovely wife and I moved to the western section of town notoriously known for its gay inhabitants. We knew it, they knew it, we all knew it. It was an absurd inside joke; my former second year dorm roommate Boy Bruce had prepared me well. I wasn't worried. No longer in the relative safety of the dental dorms, we had ventured to live in our own rented apartment. I had done so in my freshman year, but that had been a bad dream. This time I would have a decent place where my new bride would feel comfortable and secure. Hah, *Not*! The most we could afford was a miniscule, one bedroom, three story walk-up with a stinky Chinese restaurant on the bottom floor! What can I say, it's the best we could do at the time. And this was considered a real coup, according to knowledgeable friends and family. I had heard about its availability from senior dental students that were going to move out of it. During the spring of my second year, I checked it out and it seemed reasonable to live in. The surrounding neighborhood seemed okay. I didn't hear any gunshots. The streets were rather quiet; of course this was probably the case on most weekends. The dilapidated and infested building was owned by a slick, Porsche-driving orthodontist, and his two wayward sons lived in it, or so I was told. My pharmacist wife and I signed the lease that summer and left for a belated three week honeymoon trip to Florida. We would commence living as a bona fide married couple in our first apartment upon our return. My parents helped us move our scraggly stuff from the dental dorms to the apartment. Plus they had also brought hand-me-down furniture from their home that we badly needed. Multiple crosstown trips and then we were finally settled. It only took a day of effort! My parents were no longer surprised or overanxious at my living accommodations, having lived through the previous years' debacles and living arrangements. No one said a word. My wife took it all in stride. She was a brave and hard to rattle mountain girl (and still is). Adversity was not a word in her vocabulary. She was also a svelte and stunning blonde (and still is), but no prima donna. It was a place to live with her new husband, period! Maybe my future as a "Doctor" made all this palatable to my wife and parents; they never told me how they really felt. I didn't want to know. There were only two apartments per floor, so we quickly met all our quirky neighboring tenants. We also quickly learned that the building's radiator heating system worked once daily, roaches and mice were the norm, and a mysterious drug addict lived down the hall. We had roaches in our apartments in undergrad, so that didn't faze us. Mice were friendly folk that just wanted a bite to eat. The Chinese food stank didn't rankle us either. After all, we ate the stuff at least monthly. But the sudden loud rumbling noises behind our pad at all hours on weekdays did concern my wife. With train tracks virtually right behind our building, she blamed me for not knowing about the deafening sounds prior to signing the lease. It turned out that the tracks were defunct and there were no trains. Tractor trailer trucks were making those hideously obnoxious booming sounds by hitting potholes on the roads all around us. Who knew? It sounded just like trains. The landlord was reasonably decent and accommodating. He was thrilled that a "respectable" fellow dentist (not yet) that could afford the monthly rent was living in his building. One day early in our tenure he stopped by to check on his two sons and say hello to us. He told us in hushed tones to keep our eyes on his drug-addled dentist son down the hall. What? And also to keep an eye on his drug-dealing/abusing messenger-boy son on the second floor. What? I guess this was better than having them live at his home in some posh neighborhood and gumming up his social scene. This way he could keep tabs on them; at least he knew where they lived, and rent-free, for that matter. We were eventually introduced but rarely saw those two miscreants.

Of course the dentist son did sort of work at some chop shop dental clinic he owned, we were told, and he did have a nice dentist girlfriend that came for her booty call now and again. However, we kept out of his life except for very little small talk. He seemed gaunt and in dire need of rehab, as did his uneducated younger brother. All their indoor pot plants and hydroponics obviously didn't bother their old man. He wasn't about to narc on them. Maybe he was a buyer himself? A dime bag here, a dime bag there. You never know about these things. I never bought anything from them. I just wasn't in the mood for any bizarre reefer madness. I didn't trust their weed! My wife and I would lock our triple locks on our metal door and explore our neighborhood on weekends. We did the usual, restaurant adventures we could afford, plays and musicals that were cheap, and just walkabouts on the streets. It was all new and exciting for a young couple. The only thing that really chafed my wife was letting me go out by myself. It was bad enough having all the obviously gay men give me the once over in her presence, but being alone I would not stand a chance. It was a funny thought. I valiantly resisted all temptations, however, and teasingly reassured her that no man would steal my heart or private parts. Testosterone beats estrogen by a mile as far as libido goes but the neighborhood wasn't that overtly sexualized, at least not in the daytime. I remember running into a neighbor one evening near a Chinese restaurant we frequented (not the dive in our building). He had had a few too many and profoundly told us that, "We were all gay inside. Don't be afraid." I'm not sure what he meant by that. Was it a metaphor, a euphemism, a literal statement? My wife still clutched my arm tightly during our promenades around town. I was her man and she let everyone know it. Whenever I reminded her that we were all gay inside, she just scowled and laughed, a bit nervously I might add! I was never once propositioned or sexually assaulted, maybe I wasn't as good looking as my wife thought I was. I found the whole thing comical. We "survived" living in that two-bit apartment for two years before once again moving on to new lodgings.

57

Don't Step On the Crack

There were double doors on our walk-up building entrance. The first set was unlocked, but the second set had rather substantial locks. If you had no keys and wished entry, you had to be buzzed in by a tenant. Secure, right? My wife had to leave our apartment early daily for her job as a pharmacist for Pathmark Pharmacy, a large chain pharmacy enterprise. On more than one occasion she would tell me that a very disheveled and odorous bum or hobo (sometimes it's hard to tell) was sprawled out inside the second set of doors, nice and warm, comfy, and smoking crack. She would literally have to step over him to get out of the building. He seemed well nourished and harmless enough, and fully absorbed in his destructive folly. She would always say good morning to him and ask how he got inside. He would curtly reply with the same daily answer, "Don't step on the crack!" He had dozens of crack nuggets strewn about himself, and my wife had to be careful and not step on those precious pieces, lest he got angry or something. My wife didn't want any trouble at 7 o'clock in the morning, so she was careful. He was gone by the time I exited the building a few hours later, although his small crack pipe was neatly but visibly tucked away in between two mortar-less bricks. Everyone had to have seen it, but no one removed it. He and his colorful pipe disappeared after the coldest winter months had passed and we never encountered him again. We never found out how he had gained admittance inside. Maybe he was a former tenant with a key or a clever locksmith? I mean, even tramps had former jobs, I guess. Maybe someone sympathetic kept buzzing him in? Had he figured out how to live a stress-free, free-lunch kind of life, albeit drug addled? Of course mental illness could have been the replacement for a Utopian mind. Maybe I should have met him and learned something. Maybe not.

58

First Subway Ride

Locals called it the train, we called it the subway. Same thing. My wife and I avoided taking the "train" for a long time, using foot power, buses and cabs to get around in our town. We had no car (it was stowed at my parent's home); very few people did. But one fateful day, my wife was forced to take the subway to a distant locale for a mandatory pharmacy conference, as required by her employer. She had to get up extra early and figure out how to navigate the subway system. Confident of her course, she kissed me goodbye at 5 a.m. and embarked on her trek. This would be her first time buying a token and riding a train. And the first time being out and about before the crack of dawn. She was scared and so was I! This was a time before cell phones were invented, so we couldn't reach each other for comfort. And most public pay phones were usually broken. She left our apartment, took the crosstown bus to the train station, and got on. The rest is her story: The token buying and boarding were uneventful, but the rest of the ride was strictly out of a

Stephen King novel. It was cold outside, the subway car was dark and stinky, with no ventilation. Graffiti was everywhere, inside and out. Dilapidated and antiquated would be too kind to describe the car's interior. She sat down in a corner amidst four other riders. One older and disheveled man had on a trench coat, another gentleman looked ill, and a garishly made up women looked like a worn-out hooker. At least her child looked okay. The ride started out normally until the old man started to masturbate under his coat while staring at the young girl. The "ill" man was talking to himself and literally climbing the sides of the car (probably high on heroin, but who knows), and the "streetwalker" and child started to fight loudly. My wife took this all in and then remembered why we didn't take the train anywhere; her worst nightmares were confirmed and then some. My paranoia and warnings to her now made sense. At the very next stop, three young African Americans boarded and, with intimidating countenances on their faces, approached my wife. She was naively relieved to see them. Maybe they would protect her if the clowns next to her really got out of hand. After standing around for a few seconds, the black trio beat a hasty retreat to the opposite end of the train car and cowered meekly in their seats. So much for her protectors. This crazy train ride kept up until her deposit point. As she exited and looked back, the foursome were still at it and had never really acknowledged her presence. So this was what it was like riding the rails. Of course, later, when she confided this story to local friends, no one believed her. It had been an aberration but a lasting memory that she still hasn't forgotten. Maybe it was the time of day, maybe it was just bad luck. At least she had arrived at her destination unscathed physically. Mentally, who knows? The train ride back home that evening was more peaceful, she said rather cavalierly. Just some panhandlers, a few bums, a few religious "nuts," a few "thugs" and a cop were present in her car. She was no longer a newbie rider! I was next.

59

That Squirrel Looks Funny

As poor newlyweds, my wife and I liberally partook in any and all free entertainment in the town we lived in. By third year, my maddening and exhausting scholastic schedule had eased off a bit allowing me some extra time to spend in recreation. Walking to the local park became a weekly excursion. It was good, clean fun. However, you had to leave by sundown otherwise you risked being accosted by the "bad element." Weekends were ideal. There were ice cream and Italian ice vendors, new mothers with strollers galore, and us newbies. There was also plenty of animal life around including birds, chipmunks, mice, and squirrels. We both loved nature and greatly enjoyed our strolls to this delightful piece of grassed wild kingdom. My wife loved feeding the critters, especially squirrels. One time, she began throwing snacks to a very tame gray squirrel sitting on its haunches, begging her for more chocolate morsels. She couldn't believe how friendly it was; and sitting so close to us, as well. I grew suspicious when I noticed the hairless tail curled neatly behind its back. I chuckled and whispered to my wife that she was in fact feeding a large rat. She recoiled a bit in disbelief but then continued unfazed as a food purveyor. Hey, the park was our version of a mini zoo and rat or not we were determined to enjoy ourselves! Besides, after dodging black bears, moose and coyotes while growing up in upstate New York, a little rat wasn't going to intimidate my wife. Mountain folk were undeterred by pests or pan handlers. Bring 'em on!

60

The Break-In

Our solid steel door had three deadbolt locks on it, and we were still robbed! There was a Medeco, a magnetic MIWA, a Schlage, and an interior lock-bar metal door rod connected to the floor, in case of trouble. This happened when I was a third year dental student and my wife was a pharmacist in town. This was the three story walk-up we lived in, owned by a rich Long Island orthodontist. We came home after a weekend visiting relatives to find trouble; the door was slightly ajar with no obvious signs of forced entry. How could this be? We *always* diligently locked up as we left; our pockets held the heavy keys to prove it. As we slowly meandered through our flat, feeling violated and vulnerable, we discovered that only one item had been stolen: my wife's $200 gold necklace. Not the cash in the top dresser drawer, not the TV or stereo components, or other jewelry, etc. Just the gold necklace. Should we file a claim with our renter's insurance? Did we even have a jewelry rider? Should we call the cops? What would they do? Dust for prints over a necklace? We both knew who did it. The only parties with keys to our place were the owner and his drug-addled dentist son, who lived down the hall and was the supposed super for the building. He always looked like he had just fallen out of a tree. I angrily knocked on his door but to no avail. He never answered it. Maybe he wasn't there. Yes, we ran into his dentist girlfriend now and again in the hallway on her way to a sexual tryst, but not him. She said he was still living there and didn't understand what all the fuss was about. My wife would check the girlfriend's neckline for her necklace at these meetings, but no dice. We told the landlord that we suspected his son. No response. We ended up changing one lock and mailing the spare key only to the millionaire landlord. We moved out two years later with no more break-ins but with the mystery unsolved. The super/doper/dentist was eventually forcibly removed by family members and briefly hospitalized for unspecified drug abuse. Duh!! We finally did run into him briefly just before moving out. He was a changed man. He had gained weight and looked respectable, as a dentist should. However, he feigned ignorance and astonishment; he remembered nothing, knew nothing, and was rather curt and dismissive. End of story. Somewhere, some lady is wearing my wife's gold necklace, all for a dime bag or some blow.

61

Lack of Attendance?

By third year many classes started to suffer from student absenteeism and our school took notice. It was nothing new, however, but the dental college was determined to finally put its foot down and make an example of our class. Therefore, each lecture would be videotaped at the start and later reviewed and students counted. Was it an invasion of privacy? Was it legal to do? No one said anything. I mean, the school was busy crushing Walkmans right and left because of a Messianic zeal to obliterate personal freedoms; why was this any different? The administration had previously and futilely tried sign-in sheets (which ended up being doctored); the honor system (yeah, right); roll calls (I didn't know we had such talented ventriloquists in our class; Jeff Dunham move over); hand raises (the Mets could have used all the switch hitters in our class; students alternated raising their hands upon being called upon to cover for absent brethren); and required sign-out signatures (so that's where doctors get that illegible writing from). All these attendance programs had failed. The videographic solution finally hooked us, or did it? Gee, the cameras started to mysteriously malfunction a few days into the experiment. What the hell? Videotapes popping out of the machines, cut cords, loose wires, gum mysteriously lodged in the wall receptacles? The school got the message. Hey, if we didn't want to learn, it was our business, right? If a patient got the wrong tooth pulled, whose fault was it? That was the rub. Whose job was it to be ultimately responsible for us dental learners? Students, the college of dentistry, the state education department? The state licensing boards examined minimal competency, that's all. If you passed, you were a dentist, ready to practice. So what if you missed the classes on shade matching and antibiotic prescribing? Oh well. Even though I was in a light sleep through most of the lectures, I managed to attend all of them. Somehow I learned and retained most of the required dental knowledge. I purposely had feigned narcolepsy in many a class, probably much to the chagrin of classmates and professors alike. But at least my body was present and accounted for!

62

I'm Estonian, Too

I was born in the U.S.A. to Estonian immigrant parents, both of whom became white collar professionals and succeeded at the American dream. That's what I spilled out when pressed by the hawkish chairman of the Removable Prosthodontics department, Dr. Z. W. Nicholas. I had previously set up an after school meeting with him by way of his mean and often obstinate secretary. This was the same bespeckled and lab coat attired bitch that made life miserable for us peon students. I merely desired a quick meeting with the head honcho to discuss prosthodontics residency possibilities after graduation. Well, there I was, ready for sage advice from a no nonsense man. His girl Friday glared at me as I was ushered into his inner sanctum. She removed her glasses as I stumbled past her; she was better looking than I had realized. The head man looked up my grades and instantly lit up. I was O.K. in his book. The secretary then sauntered seductively into his office, bottle of scotch in hand, and smiled at me demurely as if she had a secret. She perched effortlessly on the end of his desk as if it was rehearsed. Without the lab coat and glasses, she was smokin' hot! I felt special and weird at the same time. She knew I was staring at her but she belonged to the alpha male in the room. I was offered a drink but I declined. The prof started drinking and pontificating. He knew this prosthodontist and that one; this program and that one, etc. This went on for a while. I didn't have any questions. After a few too many, both of them were literally beaming at each other. I felt awkward and creeped out. Was this the normal Friday Happy Hour? What about Shabbat? What about his wife? Wow, what a school! Then the bombshell– he practically yelled out that he was Estonian, too. What was that? "We are practically brothers," he erupted in glee. I had to leave after he put his arm around his "work wife" as she started to unbutton her top. I hope I didn't miss out on a threesome, but I doubt it. The secretary was extra nice to me the rest of that year and frequently gave me that all-knowing smile. I wasn't going to rat them out and they both knew it. I'm glad I had that "productive" talk with the chairman and bonded with him as a fellow Estonian. Could Dr. Nicholas, an Orthodox Jew, also be an Orthodox Estonian? Only at my *shul*.

63

Tell, Show, Pee

First, a shout out to all the certified pediatric dentists out there: bless you! Second, let's reminisce about the third-year's mandatory dental clinic called Pediatric Dentistry (formerly called pedodontics, or just plain pedo). This was no blessing. Inadequately staffed and very poorly run, it was a long-running painful joke for most third year dental students. The weekly clinic started at 1 p.m. Students would arrive promptly and be assigned patients at the front desk. We would then lead the small fry and parents (mostly mothers) to partitioned operatory cubicles in a large room. The cubicles were side by side. Imagine a huge room filled with sixty or more morose students and at least as many unwilling, unruly preschoolers and their parental units. Of course by 1:30 p.m. there was still no faculty present and only a few pediatric postgrad students sauntering in. Oh, did I mention that all work was graded and a certain amount of procedures were needed for graduation? Gee, no pressure there. Finally the arrogant professors arrived en masse and the agonizing process of starting actual work began. All work was first approved and signed off on by the faculty. Did I mention that 90 percent of the patients only spoke Spanish? And there were no interpreters or assistants for us lowly students. None of us spoke any Spanish, by the way. After carefully treatment planning the proposed therapy and sequence, each student stood in a long line to get a professor's start signature. At last we could begin! Oh, it was 3 p.m. by now and the clinic ended at 4 p.m. Hurry! And only needles were allowed to be used for anesthesia. No gas (nitrous oxide) or I.V. sedation was allowed as in private practice. The monster in my chair was squirming in pain and the mother was hysterically screeching at me in Spanish, "Dolor, dolor." Remember, you were being watched and graded on everything. Deportment was important. Maybe I should have employed a secret weapon; a philosophy/technique learned in the pediatric dental lecture course. Proven to work miracles, it is called Tell, Show, Do. First, you explain the procedure to the tiny tyke, then you show how it's done, and then you do it. Simple and effective, with very little language required. I listened and watched my friend in the adjacent cubicle, syringe in hand, do his best Tell, Show, Do routine in English on his unwilling child. The kid was bawling, the mother in tears, and my friend red-faced and almost crying himself. I noticed a large stain on the front of the kid's pants. Tell, Show, Do turned into Tell, Show, Pee! Simple, even a four year old would get it. *Not!* That's how the rest of the year went in Pedo Clinic.

64

The Velvet Harpoon

Although I had heard rumors of a certain malevolent removable prosthodontics professor who worked in the third year prosthodontics clinic, I never ran into him personally. And, that adage could have applied to most of the professors at my school. This story is hearsay, second hand news, but based on peer-reviewed facts. It's compelling dental school drama because it is a typical scathing example of the legalized and systematic mental abuse that was foisted on us unwitting students, even encouraged by the higher ups. Here is how it went down: All dental work to be started by a student on a patient first had to be reviewed, approved and signed off on by a clinical dental professor. To the unwary, unlucky or uninitiated, this certain professor appeared to have an unusually likeable disposition and a winsome approach to patients and students alike. He was a very jocular older dentist that seemed easygoing and was probably an easy A (all student dental work was graded). Well, the way I heard it, things always started out great and proceeded swimmingly.

No matter what kind of work was presented by the student, she/he always received an A for the particular procedure and much praise from this dentist. However, when it came time to receive an overall grade for the completed and finished procedure, the fangs would come out. This dentist would literally tear the work apart and berate the stunned and helpless student in front of all onlookers. And the final grade was usually no higher than a C. "Do it over" was his usual closing remark to the student. Everything had been velvety smooth sailing and then– *Gotcha*! Jeckyll and Hyde? Because there was always a chronic shortage of professor dentists in the clinics, most students had to continually work with this *schmuck*. Savvy students switched to other professors, but sometimes you just couldn't. He caused many of my third year peers much undeserved heartburn. Again, I never worked with that dick; his antics could have been an anomaly, perpetrated by a few bad apples. Nah, I still believe those apples to this day; he was rotten to the core!

65

Sushi Yummy

It had been an honor to be asked by a former dental row instructor to work for him part time as an assistant after school. I am still grateful to this day for that opportunity and experience. My hours were Wednesdays and Fridays, 5 to 8 p.m. The third year schedule was not as brutal as the previous two years had been, so I could swing it. Besides, my new bride was working full time so I figured I should contribute something financially to the household as well. My dental mentor was a true *mensch* in every sense of the word: hardworking, nose to the grindstone, diligent and truthful. He had that slightly paranoid, put-upon persona, but was a delight to work for. Whenever someone asked him about his practice, he would always reply, "Could be busier." It was one of those throw away lines that kept him humble, I guess. He was actually busy enough, from what I could tell. He had a ridiculously small practice in a nice downtown office building. It had only two operatories and he was literally a one man show! His was not the "million dollar" practice that we students all sought to emulate someday. A *mensch* for a *mensch* practice, but, he did make a good coin! I worked as a late night assistant, receptionist, bookkeeper, x-ray technician and confidante. I think he liked having me around to kibbitz with. He showed me real world dentistry, shortcuts, patient management techniques, business skills, etc. He was an excellent practitioner and a true friend to me. He tried hard. His patients knew it and loved him for it. One evening he casually mentioned taking me out to his favorite Japanese restaurant for sushi. My panicked thought was raw fish. I had heard of sushi before but had never sampled the "fishy" delicacy. So as not to be rude or ignorant, I agreed to our dinner date. That Friday night came too quickly. We dutifully walked a few short blocks to the place. The joint was nondescript, small, with one entrance, and a no frills business sign on the exterior. You could walk right past it without knowing it was there. Many popular establishments kept this moniker of fake secrecy. It was actually well known to die-hard sushi lovers. I was nervous. We entered and the authentically clad waitresses tittered and demurely catered to my boss. I surmised he was a frequent patron. We sat in front of the head chef, in full view of the raw bar and all the ocean's creepy crawlies and fish pieces. My edginess was obviously noticeable. The good doctor quickly ordered, in Japanese, two saki's on ice. Well, after two rounds of saki each, my culinary inhibitions vanished and it was time to order. I was famished. The sushi chef deftly timed each sampling and kept a running banter with my mentor. Yellow tail rolls, octopus with quail egg, eel with salmon roe, squid, tuna, and urchin. What a feast. A 50 dollar bill paid for it all and included the tip. We both stumbled out onto the street. He hailed a cab and bid me adieu. I decided to walk home as usual. It was about a half-hour walk for me and at 9:30 at night the streets were mostly deserted. I was still giddy with food and drink and hoped nobody would accost me in the state I was in. The occasional cab did pull alongside but I waved them off. I kept up a brisk walking pace, peering quickly into every alley, and kept my right hand firmly clutched around an authentic switchblade (I still have it) in my coat pocket. I had made this walk multiple times but was always vigilant regardless. I had no wallet, just I.D. in my shirt pocket and a "mugger roll" (a rolled up 20 dollar bill) in my pants pocket. Anything less than an armed holdup would have been met with resistance from me. Thankfully, that never occurred. Of course wearing a scuzzy down coat and carrying a small dog-eared bible in my left hand likened my visage to one of those "crazy people" you just don't want to mess with. Even a would-be mugger didn't want a hassle. It was a good charade and it seemed to have protected me. I arrived home safely and regaled my wife with sushi stories. She was stupefied by my dining bravery but soon became a sushi convert herself.

Note: My doctor mentor and employer ended up building a gigantic and hugely successful practice in another building after I had graduated. He remains a close friend to this day. Thank you Dr. B.

66

Dental Memories

My mentor and *mensch,* the dentist I worked for part time during third and fourth year, taught me many things and used to frequently comment on dental memory. He would always tell me to actually forget about the horrors of each dental day because those memories would only compound the disasters of the ensuing days. A clean slate was necessary to start each day refreshed and enthusiastic. I listened, learned and applied. It was easier said than done, especially for a conscientious dental student. Even as a lowly student I realized that medical professionals could never have an "off" day, no matter what the circumstances were. The resulting consequences could be steep. At least I could start practicing selective amnesia and better compartmentalize my life. It seemed to help. Unbeknownst to patients, I always tried my best, and still do, each and every damn day! Best effort, yes, perfectionism, perhaps. Living inside patients' mouths and ultimately taking responsibility for their oral health– no. I stopped beating myself up long ago, and this philosophy started in dental school. Everything in the universe, including teeth, tends towards entropy. Nothing we do has any lasting permanence. It just doesn't matter. Of course, try telling elderly and ornery Mrs. Jones that her failing denture cannot be adjusted any further because of bone loss and that she'll just have to live with recurring sore spots, a poor diet, and a floating lower prosthesis. See how *that* goes. Her universe is her mouth, and that's that. Entropy, shmentropy!

67

It's Raining Anesthetic

You would think that as juniors most of our student jitters
due to patient encounters would be gone; that the multitude
of hours already spent honing this craft would start paying
off. But no, no such luck. I was about to deliver a local
anesthetic to my patient when suddenly I felt like someone or
something was spritzing water on me. I stopped my injection
routine, stood up, looked around in bewilderment, and
then noticed it was coming from the cubicle next to mine.
Our cubicle modular operatories were right next to each
other; there really was no actual privacy for dental student
or patient. HIPAA laws weren't alive yet. Sometimes a faulty
air/water syringe could spring a leak. Or, maybe a trickster
student wanted to get my attention. It wasn't the sprinkler
system either. It was anesthetic solution being sprayed
unintentionally in my direction by a fellow student. I leaned
over and saw at firsthand the derelict situation unfolding.
The student had unknowingly misplaced the needle of the
syringe through the patient's cheek and was hosing me down

with anesthetic juice. He couldn't see where the end of the needle was pointing because he was busy looking into the patient's mouth. What a "maroon," as Bugs Bunny would say. The patient couldn't feel anything because his cheek was numb. I frantically but silently motioned to the student and he quickly got the point, so to speak. Neither of us told the patient what really happened. My buddy reloaded another anesthetic carpule, aimed better, and proceeded to give a proper injection. As I wiped off my glasses and sat down next to my own patient, I started muttering swearwords under my breath. My patient had an inkling that some sort of "quiet commotion" had occurred and asked me to explain. Keeping my poker face on, I just shook my head and gave an injection. What could I possibly say? Even a funny retort wouldn't be so funny. Silence was golden that afternoon.

68

Culling All Patients

Certain specific clinical requirements had to be made throughout dental school to progress to the next level, year, and graduate. You couldn't "technically" begin third year without first having completed the required fillings, dentures, root canals, etc., during your second year. And, starting during second year, the requirements were fulfilled on live patients! Most of these patients were local students, senior citizens, or the economically disadvantaged. Dental school fees were much lower than the surrounding private practice prices. The downsides for the patients were long waiting times to get in, long time periods for simple procedures, and quality and competence issues. If you got a jackass student that couldn't cut a rug, your dental work might end up suffering. But if you got lucky and were assigned a decent student, and had time to spare, oftentimes the resultant dental work was adequate and cheap, a winning combination. And the dental student would be racking up points in the requirements column. Sounds good, except for one thing: the student had to make sure that her/his patients showed up on time to the right clinic on the right day, and had money to pay the school. The dental patient/dental student assignment was on a first-come, first-served basis and arranged by the school. However, after the initial visit, all ensuing ones were the *responsibility of the student!* Did you catch that? If you were unlucky and had illiterate patients, ones without phones, incorrect phone numbers, or language barriers, etc., you were often doomed. Appointment cards were often useless and sometimes a cruel joke on the student. And, you couldn't amass more patients because the school divvied them up equally for fairness. You could only get a new patient when you finished work on a previous one. All work was signed off on by the professors so you couldn't cheat. It was a very disturbing situation for some of my buddies. Many sleepless nights were spent calling, cajoling, even paying off patients to come to the clinics and have the required dental work done. It was very, very irksome and draining. You paid all of this tuition money to be educated and sometimes it boiled down to one or two no-show patients that derailed your timely graduation. It wasn't a fair system, but no one seemed eager to correct it. Most professors actually reveled in glee, watching students squirm and panic whenever their patients didn't show up in the clinics, or didn't pay up. Oh, I forgot to mention that if a patient failed to pay for services rendered and skipped out, the student received no credit for the dental work done. My new wife watched me struggle during many evenings of my third year making furtive telephone calls to unreliable patients begging them to show up on time and have work done. Hours were spent explaining the rationale for treatment and the importance of my graduation. They were often exhausting and desperate times with no guarantee of the patient coming in at the appointed time, no matter how urgent my pleadings were. Fortunately, the majority of my patients did show up for four years and were grateful for my dentistry. Most even paid. Other students weren't so blessed. Some were held back, and some technically graduated on time but could not take the board exams until they finished that last darned filling or denture. I believe I started to lose my hair in the early '80s. I'm sure the unjustified burden of patient responsibility was part of my follicular devastation.

69

Too Retentive

I was there when it happened and, yes, it was funny. Not
for the student or patient involved, but entertaining for the
rest of us. And it lightened the tense mood of the third year
prosthodontics (dentures) clinic and gave us juicy gossip for
months, if not years to come. I still remember the event as
if it happened yesterday, actually 30 years ago to be exact.
The third year student responsible was an arrogant, brash
son of an orthodontist (his father taught part time at the
dental school). His out of whack ego was his undoing, at least
on that fateful day. It was a simple final denture insertion
on a patient by a dental student. Actually, not so simple.
You see the final insertion was a culmination of months of
painstaking work. If the denture had a tight, secure fit with
a perfect bite and esthetics, the student usually received
a high final grade; if not, failure! There was no gray area
in dentistry. Either it fit and looked good or it was a piece
of shit, and you had to start over. You also received a bad
grade. Well, this student's denture was crap because he was

a crappy student and did a crappy, slipshod job. You know the type. Seeing that the denture was literally falling out of his patient's mouth, he covertly mixed up some pink acrylic denture base material and applied it to the inside of the denture as a quick fix for this problem. He didn't call over his dental instructor because the denture was "imperfect" and a failing grade would have been given. He inserted the jury-rigged prosthesis into the patient's mouth hoping the added acrylic would solve the looseness problem. Now, this technique is used by all dentists on a regular basis when relining dentures, but was not actually taught to us at the time. There is a definite technique involved as well as certain precautions to be taken. The student paid no heed to the warning of fellow students around him and the patient didn't realize what he was doing to him. Suddenly, the patient started to howl and was literally writhing in pain while seated in the dental chair. Even his eyes were bugging out. Not a pleasant sight in a room full of other patients and students. Setting acrylic quickly heats up and can burn the mouth's soft tissues if not carefully watched and taken in and out periodically. The student looked aloof, as if this was a normal occurrence for him. He just stood there, staring at the patient in amusement. It looked as though the patient was really at fault. By then a cadre of professors had quickly gathered around the patient and were told exactly what had happened. One of the instructors tried to pull out the noxious denture but could not, try as he might. It turns out that the patient's upper bone structure was such that the denture got "locked" in place and could not be removed by hand. The patient started to gag and panic, began to swear loudly, and became combative. A bunch of instructors had to restrain him while one of them started to drill through the denture to effectively cut it in half, to remove it. Mind you, the patient was not numb, hysterical and thrashing about in the chair. However, within a few minutes a skillful instructor had deftly sectioned the denture and removed the two halves. The patient calmed down and the student got a failing grade and a stern lecture. We all secretly rejoiced because we thought an expulsion was imminent and, boy, did he have it coming. He was an asshole and deserved to be thrown out of school. It never happened. Although the student had violated many ethical and procedural rules, he was forgiven and graduated on time. It helped to be connected.

70

The S and M Show

One Italian, one Jewish. Oil and water, yin and yang, Mutt and Jeff, Oscar and Felix! Two polar opposite professors shared a closet-sized office and an even smaller desk, and they got along! But how? Some mysteries could not be readily solved. These older prosthodontics instructors were part-time faculty and unintentionally funny. And I mean funny. At least I thought so. Whenever I was in that clinic I had to remind myself that dental school was NOT humorous, although it was often difficult to do so. Dr. S. was slight, stocky, and nearsighted with a scowling approach to teaching us third year *nebbishes*. Gruff, but fair. If you had a modicum of talent he left you alone and usually gave you decent grades. If you fell short of his standards, he could be a bear. He spoke in low, measured tones, with just a touch of Yiddish mixed in. Dr. M. was burly, pudgy, with a curly mop of gray hair and a mustache that wouldn't quit! He was always full of himself and long winded; like a blustery day. One minute he would be boisterously condemning a poor student, and the next, politely but loudly discussing a complicated dental procedure with a perplexed patient. How these two mismatched office mates got along was an ongoing question, with no answers! I only worked with Dr. S. because he was a straight shooter. I didn't get along well with that pugnacious and obnoxious Dr. M. He was a bully, and just too damn loud! Nevertheless, he did have his share of student admirers. I often wondered how this unwitting comedy duo fared in their respective private practices. They were probably "normal." Here, in a school setting, it was another story. One clinic day, Dr. M. was absent and I nonchalantly (well, maliciously) started a rumor that he was quite ill and had projectile vomiting. The rumor spread rapidly, as I had hoped. At the next clinic session, anxious students confronted him inside his office and asked if he felt any better. He nearly blew his top when the term "projectile vomiting" came up. He bellowed loudly in protest that he was not sick, never was sick, and wanted to know how this whole ugly thing about him got started. Fortunately, no one fingered me. It was great to witness his overreaction. Fellow students in my camp laughed softly; Dr. S. figured out quickly that I was probably behind this brouhaha. He laughed in my direction and never said a word. My kind of prof!

71

A Bird's Eye View

Dr. M. was going on and on, pontificating and lecturing about partial dentures. He was wrong most of the time— at least according to the textbooks which only I and a few others had bothered to read. Whatever. Those morning talks from behind a broken lectern were mostly a boring waste of time anyway. Students professed to learn something and the faculty professed to teach something. Whereas, when it came time for the exams, only the students that had scrupulously reviewed old exams, and read numerous dental texts to actually learn something of value, stood a chance at receiving a decent grade. You know which camp I was in. Yet most of my classmates never learned. Knuckleheads! I tried to drown out Dr. M. with meditation, futuristic planning, faux somnolence, thinking about my hottie blondie fiancée, etc. No dice. He was an unwelcome ear worm burrowing into my learning center, dammit! Suddenly, as more denture slides appeared on the movie screen in front of us, I managed to accurately predict one of his favorite expressions, and shouted it out just before he did. To be fair, I had mimicked his unique nasal-sounding raspy voice before, behind his back of course. Nevertheless, what seemed like a psychic premonition, a revelation, might have been just plain psycho on my part! My wife prefers the latter analogy. I still love her. He had the denture slide all set up and a smirk on his face; then I yelled out in a near-perfect mimic of his voice, "Now here's a bird's-eye view." Then, as if on cue, he stated, "Now here's a bird's-eye view." The class erupted in laughter. He looked bewildered, surprised and then earnestly thought he was a funnyman; he didn't know that we were laughing at him. He was the joke! It had not been a particularly funny remark but, hey, every one counts. He tried to continue talking about partials, however, it just wasn't the same. The class was still reeling and tittering at my chutzpah. I had *gotten* that pompous bastard and was glad of it, only he didn't know it! Too bad. Now, you may think this was just a high-brow "inside" sophomoric prank, made by an elitist dental student in a posh and elite institution, that no one would "get" in the real world. Translation: it would be lost on most *mensches* out there. You may be correct in that assumption. Nevertheless, it's all I had to work with that day. Sorry.

72

The Fragile Incident

It was a "normal" removable prosthodontics clinic (dentures) session in the spring of my junior year. Suddenly, in a very loud and booming voice, Dr. M. started yelling. No need for a microphone or megaphone. Even the spiders in their corner webs felt the shouting. Standing next to a narrow sink, he held up an articulator with mounted dentures on it and hollered, "What kind of idiotic moron leaves an articulator with the word 'Fragile' written on it next to a sink where it might get bumped and broken?" Patients and students both cringed at his outburst. His diatribe became more vulgar and continued unabated for a good 15 minutes at least. We all looked around to see who the foolish jerk student was. No one came forward. This made Dr. M. go ballistic. Then the insults got heated and really nasty. Finally, a slightly frazzled senior student appeared from a back room adjacent to the clinic and nonchalantly strode forward to claim his articulator from Dr. M's grasp. "I'm surprised at you," Dr. M. lashed out. "You, of all people! You are the most talented senior in school. What were you thinking?" He then continued to alternate admonishment with praise. It was downright bipolar. The senior just stood there unruffled and waited patiently to get a word in. It seemed like a comedy routine but no one dared to laugh. Finally, the student got his chance. "Dr. M.," he said slowly and flatly, "The patient's last name is Fragile, and I intentionally put the articulator on the sink because I was washing it." The stunned look on Dr. M.'s face was priceless. He glared at all the people staring at him and simply growled, "Never mind." No apologies, no contrition. Of course we had just wasted about a half-hour of clinic time with all this hubbub. However, the spontaneous entertainment was welcome relief and almost worth the price of tuition. Almost. And it was good to see that bombastic blowhard get his!

73

Bagels and Lox

Third year lunches were still hearty pizza slices, although once in a while I got to taste something completely different. My good friend W. would occasionally invite me to his dorm room to indulge in bagels. Sure, I had eaten bagels and cream cheese before, but not these bagels. They were imported from another part of town, with exquisite chive and fennel infused high grade cream cheese (not Philly), and expensive lox, sandwiched in between the halves. If you're going to eat bagels, you got to go for the best! It was a real treat. He would impress upon me that the lox and cream cheese were imported, etc., etc. The trade-off for *noshing* on such a delicacy was helping him with homework and other school related stuff. It was a fair deal. I think my digestive tract was also happy; a momentary but welcome reprieve from a virtual daily barrage of tomato sauce and mozzarella cheese!

74

Library Dating Service?

During my third year I studied at the cramped dental school library on those nights when my new bride worked late, maybe two or three times weekly. There were adequate study carrels if you got there before 9 p.m. There were about five of us diehard study buddies, including by good friend W., that religiously crammed dentistry into our boneheads in that library until closing time (11 p.m.). I was newly married; none of my pals even had a girlfriend. It was hard to meet someone special if you had your nose to the grindstone 24/7. School was still irritating and trying in the third year and even most weekends were spent hittin' the books. During the course of the year, and on a regular basis, there appeared at least four cute female optometry students at our library. The optometry college was a few blocks away. I suspiciously and quizzically asked one of them once why they were at the dental school library this late at night. She curtly but politely replied that their library closed at 9 p.m. and ours was open for two hours more. A reasonable answer to a reasonable query. This went on for most of the year. No one kicked them out because the library staff never checked anyone's ID. You had to be a real dental *nudge* to be studying that hard and that late at night. I never once saw any fraternization or inappropriate behavior between those optometry students and any male dental student. Naturally, I did get up to go to the bathroom once in a while. So I was shocked to learn that by our senior year all four of my buds had become engaged to those four interloping female ocularists. Not only would they earn doctorates in Optometry, they would receive their "Mrs. Degrees" as well. Well played, ladies. Well played. But how?

75

Oh, The Inhumanities!

My lowest grades in all four years of dental school were in three separate courses taught by the same egotistical buffoon. He was a full professor of biostatistics and behavioral sciences, but basically full of shit. I wasn't the only one snookered by this character. It seemed that the easier the course looked, the harder the grading was, to justify its existence. All of his courses were jokes. Very easy lectures, very easy material. So easy as to make them somnolent; of course I was basically asleep in his classes anyway. I guess the class learned something, but you could never tell by the grades we received. To top it off, each student had to personally have an audience with the pompous prick in his office to receive his/her final grade (there was only one short answer/essay test per course). I received a grade in the 60's for each of his classes. In his office after his last course during third year, I just stared blankly at him as he berated and insulted me for my obvious lack of knowledge. I finally couldn't take it any longer, called him an asshole, told him

what I thought of his lack of teaching abilities, and started
to walk out. He grabbed me by the arm and I thought a
fracas would break out. Other students in the hallway had
heard our confrontation and were only too eager to join the
fray should a melee really start. Someone wisely stepped
between us at the last moment and the possibility of fisticuffs
was averted. I was really pissed off; so was he. However, he
quickly realized that the class sentiment did not side with
him and backed off. No action was ever taken against me.
I remember hearing that other students were also dismayed
with their grades and displayed their anger as I did. But in
the end the whole class took our lumps and moved on. Of
course, there were a few students that received A's in his
classes. At least that's what I heard. Maybe he started that
rumor himself?

Take a break!

SENIOR YEAR

76

Broken Moral Compass?

We should have had some type of ethics course in dental school, but we did not. It might have made some of the ethically challenged students stop and think. Or, at least, made them aware that other people, including patients, had rights and feelings, too. A New Age word that gets bantered about today is empathy, which addresses that very concept. In dental school you looked out for number one because your physical, mental and emotional well-being depended on it. School was that hard, with no let up. It was difficult to "feel" for patients when you had requirements to fulfill and grades to get. Many kids, including myself, instinctively knew right from wrong and sympathetically walked that empathetic tightrope on a daily basis. Others, not so much. Some were willfully unprincipled and morally bankrupt coming into school. You could just tell who they were. You could also tell that they would become extremely wealthy dentists someday. And that's what happened! There wasn't a *mensch* in the bunch. However, to be fair, these same unscrupulous students would have been "successful" in almost any business/profession. Just sayin'.

77

List of Courses
at PU College of Dentistry in the '80s

FIRST YEAR:

- *Biochemistry*
- *Dental Anatomy Lecture*
- *Dental Anatomy Laboratory*
- *Dental Materials Lecture*
- *Dental Materials Laboratory*
- *Gross Anatomy*
- *Behavioral Science*
- *General Histology*
- *Oral Histology*
- *Humanities*
- *Inheritance and Development*
- *Life Saving and CPR*
- *Microbiology*

- *Modular Clinic Orientation*
- *Neuroscience*
- *Operative Technique Lecture*
- *Operative Technique Laboratory*
- *Periodontics Lecture*
- *Periodontics Technique Laboratory*
- *Preventive Dental Lecture*
- *Preventive Dental Therapy*
- *Radiology Lecture*
- *Removable Prosthodontics Technique Lecture*
- *Removable Prosthodontics Laboratory*

Second Year:

- *Oral Microbiology*
- *Hospital Dentistry Lecture*
- *Occlusion*
- *Basic Medical Science*
- *Behavioral Science*
- *Dental Assistant Utilization Lecture*
- *Dental Assistant Utilization Laboratory*
- *Endodontics Lecture*
- *Pre-Clinical Endodontics (root canal)*
- *Endodontics Clinic*
- *Fixed Prosthodontics Lecture*
- *Fixed Prosthodontics Technique*
- *Fixed Prosthodontics Clinic*
- *Operative Dentistry Lecture*
- *Operative Dentistry Clinic*
- *Oral Medicine Clinic*
- *Oral Surgery Lecture*
- *Orthodontics Lecture*
- *Orthodontics Technique Laboratory*
- *Pedodontics Lecture (pediatric dentistry)*
- *Pedodontics Technique*
- *Periodontics Lecture*
- *Periodontics Clinic*
- *Pharmacology*
- *Physiology*
- *Radiology Clinic*
- *Removable Prosthodontics Lecture*
- *Oral Medicine Lecture*
- *General Pathology*
- *Oral Pathology*
- *Removable Prosthodontics Clinic*

Third Year:

- *Orthodontics Lecture*
- *Pain and Anxiety Lecture*
- *Pedodontics Lecture*
- *Periodontics Lecture*
- *Radiology Lecture*
- *Interpersonal Relationships*
- *Patient Management*
- *Cariology (study of tooth decay)*
- *Dental Assistant Utilization Clinic*
- *Endodontics Lecture*
- *Endodontics Clinic*
- *Fixed Prosthodontics Clinic*
- *Geriatric Dentistry*
- *Medicine*
- *Nutrition*
- *Occlusion*
- *Operative Dental Clinic*
- *Oral Cancer Lecture*
- *Oral Medicine Clinic*
- *Oral Medicine Lecture*
- *Oral Surgery Lecture*
- *Oral Surgery Clinic*
- *Orthodontic Seminar A*
- *Orthodontic Seminar B*
- *Pedodontics Clinic*
- *Periodontics Clinic*
- *Radiology Clinic*
- *Removable Prosthodontics Lecture*
- *Removable Prosthodontics clinic*
- *Esthetics*
- *Fixed Prosthodontics Lecture*
- *Operative Dentistry Lecture*

- *Intermittent morning seminars*
- *Local hospital rotations*
- *Mock Board Exams*
- *Working on patients all day in the senior modules and finishing requirements for graduation.*

Only the first three years were graded. Courses started and stopped, oblivious to the semester system. Some were weighted more than others. The fourth year was pass/fail, but still had clinical requirements to fulfill before graduation. If the requirements were not met, you were allowed to graduate but were not issued a diploma until all the work was completed. This meant summer school, with extra tuition payments, etc. Also, the board exams were postponed until the graduation credits were honored. One slip-up, one illness or one family emergency could derail a smart and talented student and cause severe anxiety/depression and the start of a career already behind the eight ball! It was sink or swim. We got a big dose of Republican/Conservative party ethos from day one; PU College of Dentistry was *not* a nanny state. Survival of the fittest, "junior." Welcome to the real world!

78

Are We There Yet?

It was fun "playing" dentist for the first few months of senior year. Our huge floor was called the senior modules. We each had our own cubicle. Our "own" front desk receptionist answered the clinic phone, made dental appointments and collected monies on our behalf. We had minimal supervision. It came from older dentists working part time to help us out. It was an exciting time, at least at the beginning. Then, the awful truth started to dawn on us. We really knew nothing about the real world. Everything was still basically being spoon fed to us to make it appear that we knew what we were doing. Luckily, my part-time, after-school dental gig with my mentor Dr. B. prepared me enormously. We did have minimal dental requirements that senior year, but they were easy to fulfill. What was really scary were the three sets of mock boards coming up, evenly spaced out throughout the year. We had already taken Part I, the written part. Everyone in my class passed it because it was relatively easy. If you had old board exams to study, you would have passed it because repeat questions were everywhere. The mock boards were the actual drilling, filling, periodontal and denture making practice exams– performed on *live* patients! There was also an x-ray reading and comprehensive treatment planning part. You had to pass all three sets of these mock exams to be eligible to take the real McCoy in May. That was just our school policy. Easier said than done. Many students passed two out of three. Not good enough. Many students had to stay after June, pay more tuition, repeat the mock tests, and take the real boards later in the year. What a pain in the ass. Talk about performing under pressure! But then isn't that what all dentists do day in and day out? We're like the Japanese hibachi chefs: each show has to be as perfect as possible or no return diner/patient. So, these mock exams made a mockery of the inept and unfortunate, and made the rest of us miserable but competent. Stress, stress, stress! Boy, I really enjoyed make-believe dentistry during those first few months of senior year. I hoped it was not all downhill from there. It was.

79

We're All Gay, Again

As I may have stated before, senior year in dental school was easier than the previous years. No more lectures, no more arduous studying, etc. With the exception of fulfilling obligatory clinical requirements and taking mock board exams, it was only a relatively deranged year. Working on patients as would-be dentists was still hard and full of aggravation, even then. However, at least I had extra time on weekends to take in the sounds and sights of our adopted town with my new wife. On a hot spring morning in mid-May, we were talking and walking toward the middle of town. There seemed to be music in the distance and we could sort of make out a bit of commotion going on in front of us. We questioned ourselves as to the possibility of a holiday we had missed. It looked as if a parade was going on. What could this be? A circus in town? Maybe a funky funeral procession? Quickening our steps we just had to find out what was going on. We eagerly positioned ourselves at a street corner, held hands and watched the proceedings with wide open eyes. Well, it didn't take long for the stares to start. Everyone was looking at us with condemnation and puzzlement. We felt uncomfortable and then noticed that the marching in front of us was actually a Gay Pride parade; it was never mentioned in the media, at least not the kind we read and watched. We seemed to be the only heterosexual couple in sight, and really stood out. What really gave away the parade were brightly painted signs carried by the raucous marchers, such as Delaware Dykes, etc. Embarrassed to the max, we slowly melted away to whence we came. The next day my former roommate, Boy Bruce, excitedly called me and asked if we had seen him amongst the merry revelers. He told us he joined the best looking men's group, called The Pennsylvania Penile Code, and had been wearing an orange string bikini bottom. I said, "No, we didn't see you." But we *had* seen lots of exposed parts, pieces, tits and tats that unfortunately lodged in my memory forever. I hope all those bare buttocks had sunscreen on them!

80

Of Mice and Mets

My wife had gotten used to living in our dank one bedroom walk-up on the west side of town. She was gainfully employed as a full-time pharmacist and I was in my senior year in dental school. There were no more classes to take and no more hard core studying to do. Of course there were mock board exams to take and fulfill clinical graduation requirements, but that was a far cry from the numbing and soul-leaching daily grind of the previous years. Now I could actually breathe a little. Now we could actually have a little fun. We didn't spend much on home furnishings and knickknacks because we physically did not have the room. We saved our money but did participate in many low-cost events in our surrounding area. Our apartment life was a bit congested and tight, but we were both thin; we didn't bump into each other, unless on purpose. Many warm and wonderful evenings were spent with the windows open, watching the Mets play baseball on TV. It was a magical year. I was more of a football fan, but how could anyone resist the hardscrabble Mets with their unique cast of characters– Carter, Darling, Strawberry, Gooden, Hernandez, Dykstra, Mookie, etc. The Yankees were just not an exciting baseball team at the time. The Metropolitans had the mojo going all yearlong. Many games were won in the last exciting innings, which made them the superstars of the media sports world. Yes, the G-men were good that year also, and ended up winning the Super Bowl with Simms and company. But the Mets were the darlings. My wife and I would watch the TV games and discuss the players as if we really knew them. They were that familiar. Mrs. Mouse and her brood would quietly scurry out from inside the oven and join us in front of the TV in the darkened apartment. They just sat there, close to us, unafraid, peering at the TV. Traps and poison were a waste; they didn't work. Momma mouse was too smart. If anyone had spied on us it would have been a surreal scene. Here was a human couple and a bunch of well-behaved rodents watching a baseball game on television together in the same room, some three feet apart from each other. What's wrong with that picture? It really happened. We coexisted all that year; the mouse family grew up and eventually stopped showing up, right after the Mets had won the World Series in October. Coincidence? I'll never know. It's funny what you get used to as being the norm. Dental school comes to mind.

81

Sports and Dental School

I'm not talking about alcohol, pot, sex or being a fan. I'm talking about participating in a real sport, participating and competing, participating and winning! Tennis was and is my athletic endeavor, although I throw a mean javelin, sprint short distances in masters track meets and have won international snowshoe sprint races. However, back in dental school, there just was no time, period. A few students tried to go to some university workout classes early in the first year but could not continue. I tried to get to a tennis court and maybe played twenty times in four years. Exercise for me was home weightlifting (small and light puppy weights), some push-ups and sit-ups. I played darts regularly with some fellow students in the dental dorms during second year, but I don't think that counted as a serious or strenuous sport. Some students gained weight; I lost weight. My fiancée, and then wife, told me repeatedly that I was shrinking. I think she meant my body, although she may have been referring to my naughty parts, as well. Anyway, I rededicated myself back to my sports after graduation and currently play in tennis tournaments, enter track meets, hit the gym regularly and continue to try to keep in shape. Of course round is a shape, isn't it?

82

Yitz and Rachel's Wedding

Oh *goy*, I had misplaced my emergency yarmulke! No
worries, though. I would be given a complimentary one at
the door, as I walked backwards into the hall. It was our first
Orthodox Jewish wedding and my wife and I were going
to soak in the celebration. It felt liberating indulging in a
free and extravagant evening away from dental school. We
both knew the bride and "goofball." I had known Yitz since
freshman year. He was basically a good egg; he really tried
hard. A bit of a live-wire and jokester (tough when you're
Orthodox), he personally invited us to attend his nuptials.
We knew nothing of the customs, protocols, etc. What about
the gift? We were somewhat clued in by the time the big
day arrived, however. First, we stopped at a mutual dental
student's apartment to go over last minute instructions, for
the ladies to freshen up, and to have a few frosty ones (kosher
beer). We had our cash wedding present; we were ready!
It was a blast. Everyone had a great time. It didn't matter
that my wife's dress was dark blue instead of the mandatory

dark black. And it didn't matter that the dancing was done in sexually segregated circles– men with men, women with women. At least my wife and I got to eat dinner together. We remarked at the vigor and enthusiasm shown by the out-of-shape adults going nuts on the dance floors. No one suffered an MI afterwards, I hope. Yitz was beaming and sweating, Rachel was demurely smiling while tugging at that damned itchy, jet black wig she was wearing. We ate, we partied, we went home spent. It had been a wonderful Saturday night that I will not soon forget. I hope you guys are still married.

83

DDS or DDE?

Sometimes I wondered what kind of degree I was getting. Was it a Doctor of Dental Surgery or a Doctor of Dental Entertainment. Maybe a dual degree? Three long years of mental torture had really brought out my twisted sense of humor, most likely as a coping mechanism. To ease the pain some students drank to excess, some smoked to excess, some probably even masturbated to…. I cracked people up to excess, or at least I tried to. After all, isn't every patient encounter performance art, with a bit of science thrown in? As mentioned before, we were trained to be similar to hibachi chefs: they appear out of nowhere, do their incredibly skillful routine, bow, and leave for the next table. That's how I felt as a dental student going into my senior year, and still do. Aren't we just highly paid and skilled professional entertainers that happen to need malpractice insurance? I don't know. I never took myself too seriously in dental college and neither did most of my patients. Even so, most dental school patients returned time and again for my "act." Ditto in private practice. Although way over the top, maybe Patch Adams was onto something?

84

The Horror of Movie Night

I was not in student government. And I wasn't in any
fraternity, or sorority either. I prided myself as being a GDI–
God Damn Independent! Nevertheless, when mandatory
"school sanctioned" policy called for student activities
to help rejuvenate and relax us, the elected class officers
and student frat officials usually came groveling to me for
guidance. Why me? Did I really have the same "reputation"
here as I did in pharmacy college? I guess so. Just when you
thought you weren't fun anymore, some droll sad sack dental
student cozies up to you and begs for some "fun" advice.
Fuck them! None of these administration-suck-up rat fink
bastards and shills cared for me personally, and vice versa.
We basically tolerated each other. They wanted to be cool, I
was coolly ambivalent. Anyway, this time I was cajoled into
suggesting an amusing and lively movie for movie night, a
new distraction to be held monthly in the main auditorium,
just for our senior class. I looked squarely into the pudgy
and pathetic face of our class vice president and said, "Rocky

Horror Picture Show." Of course, she had never heard of it, and I figured as much. The film had only been out for ten years and played to huge audiences around the country. This sheltered and snooty "JAP" wouldn't have known the difference between *Rocky Horror* and *Debbie Does Dallas*. Her naïve, all-girl selection committee unanimously approved the flick, as did the administration higher-ups, and we were all set for movie night. It was a cunning plan and I could hardly wait. Quick history update: *Rocky Horror Picture Show* originally debuted on stage as a raunchy, campy, sci-fi horror musical in the early '70s. A subsequent B-movie was made (with future big name stars) and it quickly morphed into a cult classic. The music-oriented, kinky, transvestite-themed film with burlesque overtones became a staple event during midnight showings at designated theaters throughout the U.S. Many theater-goers came dressed up as the actors and mimed their actions from the movie screen. I had started as a "virgin" at my first showing and then must have attended at least twenty or more subsequent shows as an undergrad in pharmacy college. Oh, did I mention that bringing props was a must? I walked into the large darkened lecture hall a few minutes prior to the movie start on that Saturday night clutching two large brown paper bags full of "stuff." Sitting down next to my good buddy W. in the back row (where I normally sat during dental lectures), I proceeded to carefully pull out an assortment of obtuse objects from the bags, much to the jaw-dropping amazement of my classmates sitting all around us. A large squirt gun super-soaker, slices of toasted bread, bags of white rice, Scott's brand toilet paper rolls, and newspaper. Why? What was going to happen? And why was I talking to the screen out loud during the opening credits? The *Rocky Horror* learning curve was steep, however, some of the students finally started to get the gist of the evening. They realized that this was more than a film to watch; it was a comedic interactive event and I was the narrator/instigator. I didn't remember all the obligatory lines (watch that thumb, Riff Raff; picky picky picky, is that any way to pick your friends? What, meatloaf again? etc., etc.) and flubbed many obvious puns. I did the best I could. After throwing rice at everyone during the onscreen wedding ceremony, squirting cold water everywhere during the raining scenes, launching toilet paper and toast at the screen at the appropriate times, most of the class finally "got it." Near the movie's end, people actually started to laugh at my narration-interaction with the onscreen actors. Things were going as planned. I glanced over at the class V.P. and her cohorts. They sat there cowering and horror-stricken, picking rice out of wet hairdos. This horror movie was definitely not what they imagined it would be. It was filthy, R-rated, low brow, and most unintellectual, kind of like WWE Championship Wrestling. I loved it! The auditorium seats and floor were a mess, covered with wet rice, wet newspapers and soggy toilet paper. The lights went on and I got steely stares from the girly-girl committee. It was priceless. I had thoroughly hoodwinked them. They had been snookered, bushwhacked! The administration roundly admonished them for the inappropriate film selection and ensuing shenanigans that transpired in the assembly hall that night. The cleanup alone turned out to be very arduous. I was never asked for my opinion about student activities again; movie night was officially scrapped. Good! It served those goofy, goody-girlies right. Maybe they would finally grow up? Perhaps it was me that needed to mature? Nah, Clowns-"Я"-Us was my unofficial moniker, and still is.

85

Dentistry, Drinking, Divorce, and Death

It seems that dentistry has always had a nasty reputation as a profession with a high divorce rate, high suicide rate, and rampant alcoholism. I have no statistics to either confirm or refute those claims. They were all hearsay and throwaway statements in the early '80s, when I was in dental school. Were they true, or at least based on facts? It was hard to tell. The media was convinced it was so. I will tell you from personal experience that many male dental students were in it for the money, power and women. Whether character traits such as greed, megalomania and lust of incoming students in fact predicted their futures was difficult to ascertain. We students had many seemingly harmless and idle discussions about Porsches, hot women and owning a chain of dental offices. I'm sure many professionals in other fields had similar discussions. Nevertheless, when expectations were not met, that's when problems arose. Even in school there was the uptick of alcohol consumption among certain frustrated and agitated students. There were also some marriage breakups. Wasn't this the societal norm, though? Or was it unique to dental students and dentists? Maybe I was one of the lucky ones. I'm still here; I don't own a Porsche (classic Corvette, instead) or a dental chain (I invested in real estate, instead), but confess to hoisting a few suds when my hottie blondie wife isn't looking! Today, dentistry is near the top in popularity as far as professions for students to go into. Go figure. Maybe the angst is finally gone. Maybe it's because the majority of dental students and future graduates are women?

86

Disability?

Now, I'm not against legitimate disability services. Disability services are now mainstream and readily available to those deserving of it. There, I said it. *deserving of it.* In the late afternoon of the first day of dental school we were led into a large auditorium and "tested" to determine if we had any learning disabilities. We looked at each other in frozen fear. No one wanted to be labeled as inferior and bounced out of school. This must've been a trap of some kind, or was it? The room darkened, the test packets were distributed and the lecturer started to drone on about the exam. We had to write our names and social security numbers on the answer paper. That did it. They would now know who the dumbbells were. Nothing was said about this test helping us or why it was being conducted. It was just some part of a "study" done by a certain professor with an interest in dyslexia. But then why put our names on the tests? No answer. Well, different letters, words and phrases appeared on the large screen behind the prof and we had to write down what we saw as best we could. Obviously, if you were genuinely dyslexic, it would be rough going, and maybe there would be mixed up letters and words on your answer paper as proof of your learning disability. I never heard of the results being released so I surmised that I had passed the test. And, seemingly, no students were instantly dismissed either. I never gave it a second thought until graduation day. One of my buddies came up to me after the ceremony and laughed that he got into the same prestigious residency program as me due to that long ago "dyslexia test." He proceeded to tell me, quite jovially, that he was in the know and purposely failed it badly to get extra time on exams for the duration of the four years of dental school. Only the professors knew about these "certain disabled students." Of course, some were actually learning-challenged, I presume. I proceeded to call him every bad name I could think of but then relented and called him "smart." He said that he was told ahead of time by people he couldn't name that it wasn't cheating, just getting a leg up on the competition. Now, why didn't someone educate me? When I asked my friend if maybe he really was a bit handicapped, he snarkily replied that when it came to women, he was, but not in the classroom! Is honesty really the best policy? Does my friend bill for two fillings when he only does one? Dishonesty training started early for some. It makes you wonder why some people distrust dentists.

87

Jaded Altruism

As senior dental students we were forced to participate
in a few "outreach" programs for disadvantaged youths
and indigent seniors during the year. It amounted to a few
extremely stressful and exhausting hours here and there at
various health/medical locations in town. They were set up by
our college and were just exams and screenings, nothing too
complicated. The need was great, the resources scarce. I guess
we were involved to help foster some type of empathy in us
and to help our fellow man without regard to compensation.
We never looked into it with deep psychological thought,
however. Sure, we received a bit of gratitude in Spanish, and,
sure it made some of us feel warm and fuzzy all over. However, did we really achieve anything substantial? We quickly
realized that we could have been working 24/7 and the line
of desperate and needy people would never end. Why do
those retired and goody-two-shoes dentists featured in dental
magazines travel abroad to have their egos stroked by treating
foreigners for free when they could set up a "dental tent" in

any large American city and be swamped? I thought charity begins at home, but there's no glory in that, is there? Many so-called dental scholars complain that caries and dental needs are rampant in poverty-stricken areas, usually without a dentist in sight. Unfortunately, most dentists cannot work for free for long, unless they are retired or somehow being subsidized. Free dentistry won't pay for the Benz or school loans. However, there is no access to care problem; there is an access to cash problem, especially in the poor areas of many countries, including ours. If every person in an impoverished area won the lottery, a slew of dentists would magically materialize overnight and set up shop. That's human nature, and the nature of business! What can I say? But every patient and every mouth counts, even international ones, and if just one person gets a shot at being pain free, volunteer programs would seem successful. Anyhow, who am I to judge other dentists and their real motives? As a student those "outreaches" were overwhelming at times. And they seem to have had a paradoxically opposite long-term effect on me and most of my former classmates. In a line from the movie Meatballs, "It just doesn't matter." Maybe it does, it's hard to say. Remember, these are just my observations and opinions.

88

The Naming Game

It was always interesting to see dental school donors' names emblazoned on plaques which were in turn riveted to armchairs in the auditorium, on classroom doors, in laboratories, on the sides of cubicles, etc. I guess if you're going to donate a sum of money you should at least get your name on something. At our school, it had become ridiculous at times. During my four years, the name of the main auditorium, the name of the entry foyer, and the actual name of the school changed. The newest and largest contributor trumped the old one. No one batted an eye. The college sold out to money, mainly alumni dough. And these "name boards" were everywhere, and I mean everywhere. I often joked that if I ever sent in a donation to my dental school during a moment of weakness, I would want the large men's room in the front foyer named after me. Of course, I would be flushed as soon as a greater sum came in for the same shitter. Oh well, so far, no moments of weakness.

89

Hairline Hijinks

My hottie blondie girlfriend used to love running her hands through my long black locks, sometimes even putting my hair in a ponytail. Now, as my old lady, she runs her hands over my head of bone and complains of getting stubble-burn! What happened? All the older males in my family had luxurious pates of hair; hirsute domes were the norm. However, I started to lose it in dental school. Coincidence? I can't tell for sure. Although the length kept inching upwards toward my collar with each succeeding year of pharmacy college, it plainly started to fall out in dental school. Was it the stress, the tests, the patients, the bullshit? All of the above? At graduation I had thinning hair that at least covered most of my skull. It was all a slippery slope from there. I currently look like an old man. Oh, wait a minute, I am one! If I didn't suffer from O.L.D., I'd really be worried. But, hey, at least I can finally grow a beard, and my wife likes that!

90

Best Friends Forever Bullshit

Yeah, right! We signed each others yearbooks, gave hugs and kisses and professed in front of witnesses to stay connected. Bullshit. It had been four years of hell (well, there were a few rays of heaven thrown in) and we were all just glad to get out. Graduates were so giddy that we said things to each other that had no meaning, no relevance, and were basically party line pablum. Sure there were a few reunion parties that were poorly attended. And, sure, some dental chuckleheads ended up practicing in close proximity to each other. However, the rest of us never really bonded, and never would. Maybe it was a dental thing? You know, solo territorial gamesmanship. Maybe group practice physicians get along better? Thirty-plus years ago my best friend W. and I swore to keep in touch– I send him Happy Hanukkah greeting cards, he sends me Christian cards for Christmas. And that's it. We communicate once yearly to "keep in touch." Pathetic and sad is what it is. Is the cutthroat culture of dental school revisited forever upon its graduates? Apparently so. But wait, maybe they're all on Facebook and Twitter? Maybe I should sign up, "friend" my former friends and "tweet" those twits. Nah, that would be too easy. Wait, perhaps they're all on Tinder and Grindr, instead?

91

A Panoply of Talent?

We had them all, in spades. Old, young, male, female, LGBTQ, and more. I always assumed the medical fields were composed of old white men, at least that's who my family and I went to back in the day. Well, things really changed by the time I became a dental student. I don't think our class had a prototypical student. Besides being armed with various personalities, characteristics, colors and creeds, most of my cohorts also hailed from disparate and sometimes weird previous occupations. Is that why they were selected for dental school? Is that why I was selected? Where were all the bio and chem majors that came straight out of undergrad?

Here is a partial list of the eclectic, eccentric and oddball pre-dental professions/jobs that some of my classmates had prior to enrolling:

- Ph.D. in neuroscience
- Dental Lab Technician
  (actually, two of them, and boy were they gifted.)
- Ph.D. in biochemistry
- Bartender
- Accountant
- Delivery driver for the Arnold Bread Company
- Lifeguard
- Pharmacist
- Israeli commando
- ANC revolutionary in South Africa
- High School biology teacher
- Rabbi
- Truck driver
- Professional musician
- Dentist in Moldova
- Dentist in Guadalupe
- Social worker
- Chinese paratrooper
- Stripper/porn star

Great list, huh? Obviously all the incoming freshmen dental students did finish their undergrad degrees in some type of science although few immediately stepped into dental school. Some had strayed rather far from the medical field; some even ended up in deep left field before making a U-turn to dental college. By the way, we did have our requisite bio and chem majors, although they too had interesting talents. Dental school was a mismatch and clash of cultures, races, religions, ages, sexes, IQ's, etc. Perhaps that's why I fit in?

92

Senior Talent Night

I knew we had some talented people in our class, not in dentistry mind you, but in other fields. Senior Talent Night was a relatively new endeavor organized by the "authority" administration to foment some type of cohesiveness and relaxation among us grunts prior to graduation. Maybe we would be brainwashed overnight into thinking what a joyous place this had been and start writing checks to the alumni association. See, "PU College of Dentistry really cares about its students." That cleverly concealed cynical concept didn't jibe with me. Although, I must say, that night was a real eye-opener. I didn't realize how many students had put aside extraordinary talents and skills in all sorts of fields, just to pursue a guaranteed dental buck. The musicians alone stole the show. Wow! Were my classmates wise to forgo nebulous artistic dreams for a paycheck or were they second-rate wannabe hacks and really not that good? It didn't matter. At least I was impressed, and that's not easy to do– as my kids will attest. I sat there in the packed audience transfixed, as students bared their souls and showed their authentic selves. It was a true awakening for all of us in attendance. These were the same awkward and "dentally inept" folks I had poked fun at for four years. Maybe with different career choices they wouldn't have seemed so misplaced. I would have respected them as artistes; dentists, not so much. It became shamefully and blatantly apparent that dentistry would never supplant or fully dash the underlying desires of those fellow classmates on stage; it would only be a job for them, and a rather ugly one at that. How sad.

93

The Residency Shuffle

Residencies were not required of recent dental graduates in the early '80s. Most students took the board exams at the end of senior year, got their shingles, and hung them out as soon as possible. However, some of us seniors that wished to specialize or just get in an extra year of "practice" before the real practice started, looked to secure limited spots in paid dental residency programs, throughout the country. Unlike mandated medical residencies, the general dental programs were optional. Most were in hospitals; a few were dental school-based. About 30 percent of my class vied for those coveted residency berths. And we were also competing against senior dental students from the entire nation. It was a difficult and anguishing time, trying to finish up school, take the final board exams and navigate the residency applications and interview process. Our school did help us a bit and former students who were now residents gave us feedback, too. Like with most organizations looking to hire, usually the best and the brightest were selected first. The top flight residencies usually hired the top notch graduates. After multiple interviews and offers, I selected a federal government hospital dental residency position which was considered a stellar and highly ranked program, on a national basis. I had hit the big time! All that studying and sacrifice had paid off. I would be a dental resident in a very prestigious institution while making a decent coin, at least by residency standards. I ended up staying three years and completed a prosthodontic master's degree, as well. The dental residency shuffle was well worth it for me– no regrets. Although there was an embarrassing incident during this whole process that stuck with me for years in private practice. I thought it was a minor humorous blip; some people can be so sensitive. I guess I'm also included in that bunch, at times. And it was all my fault! During the throes of ecstasy upon being accepted to a highly ranked residency, I suddenly had the urge and hubris to contact a certain program that had NOT granted me an interview or even responded in any way to my application. This was at an average hospital program in the town I wished to practice in some day. It would have been nice to at least interview there, visit the area in general, and then kindly decline the offer. I was feeling cocky and quite cheeky when I fatefully decided to phone them. It didn't go well. First, I queried the secretary; she coldly answered that my application was indeed received and patched me through to the assistant dental director. I told him emphatically that

I felt insulted by not being granted an interview in light of my outstanding credentials and that I had been accepted to many great programs. He coolly shot back, "We didn't feel you would be appropriate for our program!" What the hell did that mean? I slowly exploded inside and asked him if that meant I was overqualified? "No, just not a good fit," he retorted sarcastically. In a loud and obnoxious voice I proceeded to tell him that I would have definitely accepted a job at his place had I been offered one (I was lying, of course), since I had lived in this town as an undergrad and sought to return there to practice (this was true). We argued for another five minutes and I should have let things go. But no, I decided to go for the spinebuster. I was having too much fun. Then, I dismissively uttered, "Well, doctor, you have a B program at best; I'm glad I'm going somewhere else." The shit hit the fan. He swore at me for that incendiary remark and we mutually hung up on each other. I had a hearty chuckle after that testy phone exchange and laughed some more when I told my wife later that evening. Nevertheless, that flippant and derisive diatribe haunted me throughout my early dental career when I returned to that town as a dentist. My brief loss of sanity and wisdom was all it took for the local dentists to take umbrage. Who knew how fast word would spread? Who knew that most of the local dentists finished that particular residency program? Who knew they would all hold a prolonged grudge against me for years to come? Someone in the program had not wanted me there in the first place– a spiteful and envious former graduate of my dental school, perhaps? I had my suspicions, but never bothered to find out. This town was a close-knit hive of similarly trained dentists. Outsiders were not very welcome. And here I went and called their beloved hospital dental residency program "garbage." How dare I? Such impudence. I set up shop in their midst anyway. After seven years of success in this town I relocated my private practice to an even more lucrative location in a neighboring municipality and left all those B players behind. It's funny, some of them don't speak to me to this day. Fuck them! Did I regret being so glib to that dental director in a moment of honesty? You know the answer to that one!

94

The Infamous Glue Job

Maybe he just panicked or maybe he was just a corrupt, inept, self-entitled, arrogant asshole. We all thought the latter. And, he got what he deserved, finally! It was board exam day, just before graduation. We were all perplexed and anxious, huddled in our cubicles like doomed rats. I was busy and nervously completing the afternoon operative portion on a very patient and good-natured patient– drilling and filling– and progressing along fine when I heard a loud commotion at the opposite end of the large senior module we were in. It was a very heated discussion between an elderly dental board examiner and this student in question. Of course we all stopped and stood up to get a better view of the hubbub. However, most of us were too far away to know what was going down. The anticipated fracas never occurred and we went back to the old grind. It was only much later, after graduation, that rumors started to float around that this particular student, and son of two distinguished faculty members, actually tried to cheat his way to a passing grade on the operative part of the exam. That boisterous exchange we had witnessed was the tip of the iceberg. We didn't realize that although he graduated with our class, and looked smug during the ceremony, he in fact failed that part of the boards and was precluded from taking it again for a whole year, as punishment by the State Education Department (the department that issues licenses for professionals). Wow, what a strong demerit. What did he do exactly to so infuriate the state? Again, rumor had it (there were surrounding witnesses who supposedly saw the whole thing) that after drilling too deeply into his board tooth, he tried to cover up his mistake by using Krazy Glue. You see, if the nerve gets exposed by drilling too deeply, the tooth then needs to have a root canal procedure done. All he had to have done was tell the examiner that the decay was so deep that he had no choice but to drill down after it and therefore exposed the nerve. The examiner would then ask the student if he had another tooth to work on, etc. In other words, you would get a second chance, if you had the time. Instead, he coated over the exposed and bleeding part of the nerve and had the "nerve" to call over the examiner for approval before placing the final gold filling (yes, we had to use 24 carat dead-soft gold in one part of the operative exam). The board examiner saw the red blood under the layer of glue and repeatedly poked at it, until it came out and hit a student in an adjacent cubicle. Meanwhile, the patient being numb was unaware of the monkeyshines transpiring in his mouth. The examiner and the student then got into a shouting match, with the state winning. No punishment was doled out by my school to the student and he eventually retook that exam portion and passed. However, I cringe to this day at his "entitled" behavior, flouting authority and even sassing a deputy. What would have happened in the Old West, a shootout with the Marshall? In the 1980s no such luck; only a token slap on his drillin' hand. I heard he is practicing with mommy and daddy in their million dollar private practice. Practicing is a good word for that spoiled brat.

95

The Real McCoy

All the senior class had successfully passed Part I of the dental boards and most students had passed the three sets of mock boards to be eligible for the real thing in May. Some students could not take Part II because of lack of third and second year requirements; some were recused because of failure of one or more of the mock exams. Our school was tough and strict, what can I say? The dental board exam (Part II) was a two day affair, comprised of x-ray reading, comprehensive treatment planning, periodontal therapy on a patient, fillings and gold foil on a patient, and denture making on a patient. All on real people, and all graded by humorless dentists (elderly and dastardly board members) from out of town. You know the type, the kind that tries hard to be your friend and then fails you with gusto and *relish*. We were warned about possible antics by the board examiners and dulled our #23 explorer tips just to be on the safe side (dull tips can't stick into carious tooth structure as easily as sharp points). Nobody wanted to get snookered by the fake geniality of those bastards or be blindsided by their over-aggressive "finding" of decay that really wasn't there. Failure of the boards or a part of them meant retaking that part or all parts later in the summer, or the following year. You would be out of school, had to procure your own patients, stay sharp in the meantime, pay an extra fee to use the school, keep your apartment rental lease going in town, etc. It was a real pain in the ass to fail. The school no longer helped you after you graduated. It was up to you to pass; that's why the first time was the best time, period! I remember hearing stories of students that had retaken the boards multiple times after failing the first one not because of being incompetent or apprehensive, but because of the often exasperating and unlucky circumstances that ended up befalling them during that fateful exam. OK, so the clinical day arrived. I had made the requisite patient phone calls the night before. All agreed to show up and sit for me. I admit to having been a bit nervous, but not as wired as I had been for the pharmacy boards years earlier. Passing those damn pharmacy board exams, especially the lab portion, was no picnic. Hopefully this would be easier? I had some confidence since I had aced the three mock boards. However, this was the real deal. It was Hammertime! I confidently strode into the senior module, unpacked all my necessary armamentarium (I love that word), unlocked my dental cabinets, arranged my instruments, and sat in a corner of the cubicle, awaiting my first board patient. I was a little wound up, who wouldn't be? The clock on the wall showed 8:05. And then in walked my 86 year old denture patient, Mr. P. He was beaming and excited because he was going to get a brand new and free upper denture out of this "board" experience. I had been prepping and working on him for close to six months and had previously used him for my three mock board exams. It was "legal" to utilize the same denture patient multiple times when practicing for the real McCoy. I had passed each mock test before, therefore the real one should have been a piece of cake. It wasn't. Mr. P. sat down in the chair, we exchanged pleasantries, and he dutifully opened his cake-hole. Shit! Panic time! He forgot to wear his lower denture! Although we were only making an upper denture, the lower one was vitally needed for a proper bite. Holy crapola, how was I going to do this? The patient was very apologetic and distraught. He understood the dilemma, bolted out of the chair, dashed past a bored (pun alert) examiner and ran wildly into the streets. He had no car. Great. Of course the ancient looking examiner instantly hobbled over to me and got right in my face, like an un-amused drill sergeant. He asked me what the hell was going on? I told him the truth and implored him to give me more time before I started; that I was pretty quick and should finish on schedule. He glared at me and snarled, "Quickness doesn't make a good dentist. Your patient better be here by

8:30 or I will *personally* flunk you!" I recoiled in disbelief. Wow, at least he would personally fail me and not pawn me off on some flunky. Lucky me! Many, many tense minutes passed. What could I do? That helpless feeling of doom felt horrible. Against all odds, Mr. P. promptly appeared back in my chair at 8:29, out of breath and perspiring profusely, but with a smile on his face, and with his danged lower denture in hand. The "mean" examiner passed me with high grades, shook his head and cackled, "Sonny boy, you did it. How do you feel now?" "You know how I feel, asshole," I quietly whispered to myself. My adrenaline was still pumping from the morning debacle and it was difficult to relax at that moment. The afternoon periodontics (gum work) portion should have been a breeze, or so I mistakenly thought. The patient arrived on time and was seated. All I had to do was clean the tartar and plaque from his teeth. His x-rays revealed lots of deep calculus (tartar) ringing most of the roots of the teeth. Remove it and pass, right? Not so fast, *not so fast*, bucko! The perio board examiner repeatedly poked and prodded the gums of my patient until they bled, as if searching for something he had lost. I started to become concerned when he stopped, looked up at me with soul-less eyes and spewed, "This is goddamn perio disease, very deep, very serious. A cleaning won't do. Do you have another patient you can use?" Sure, I had one in my back pocket, just in case. *"WTF?"* This patient had been approved by one of my seasoned and respected periodontics instructors. Now what was I to do? I had to think fast. If I invoked my perio professor, it would impute the examiner's judgement, not a formula for success. I said meekly, "Doctor, I will scale and root plane the lower two quadrants as preparation for the possibility of future perio surgery pending a re-evaluation in a few weeks." He scowled at me and growled, "Good answer *doctor*. I like you. You have balls to talk back to a board examiner. Go ahead." I got the green light and took off. I scraped, chiseled and debrided like a madman. The examiner was duly impressed; I passed and the patient was scheduled for a perio evaluation in a few weeks with a rising senior. Day one was mercifully over. I don't remember eating or sleeping that night. Tomorrow was the last day of the practical part of the exams. It would be the operative portion, drilling and filling. My wife was up early and left for work by 7 a.m. I scrambled to get my shit together for another grueling day. The morning patient came on time and we began the dance all over again. The a.m. session consisted of the placement of a gold foil filling in a tooth that had a cavity adjacent to the gum line. We had practiced this archaic procedure many times throughout the senior year; it was just not done any more in real world dentistry. The dental board kept it in the examination because it "tested" many skills a dentist should have mastered during the dental college tenure. It was a very challenging, exacting procedure. You had to manipulate tiny pieces of malleable 24K gold into a small cavity with special instruments and polish the filling to a high luster. It was a long, exhausting endeavor for both patient and student doctor. I finished this part uneventfully, got graded fairly, and passed. So far, so good. One more session to go; a simple filling on an upper bicuspid in a lovely female nursing student. After the anesthesia, I prepared the two-surface cavity correctly, got it signed off, and filled it with an amalgam restoration. I polished it to a gleaming shine, called over the jovial and rotund examiner who previously checked it, and presented for a final grade. He waddled over rather casually and his unwieldy frame made an audible thud in my chair as he sat down hard. He meticulously examined my work and, in between praiseful platitudes, carefully considered the filling from all angles. And then, in a flash of quickness that startled my patient and me, this behemoth roughly grabbed her head in one hand and clutched her jaw with the other. I thought he was about to kiss her! No, in one lightning fast move, he deliberately slammed her lower jaw against the upper one, and then quickly peered into her mouth. He was checking to see if my "gorgeous" (his words, not mine) filling had cracked. If it had– instant failure! Nobody had prepared me for this particular testing of occlusion. It was barbaric, though effective. He relaxed his meaty holds on the hapless patient, swiveled to me and murmured, "I almost gotcha, damn it, but didn't. You pass."

What a nice jerk. Where did these guys come from, anyway? My eyes were still bugged out; I was unnerved, which pissed me off. My poor patient was speechless and just sat there massaging her jaw. Was she just assaulted? I managed to calm myself before apologizing to her, on his behalf. She nodded and we parted company. I had passed the Northeast Regional Boards and would soon be a real dentist. Wait, what was that same patient doing in my chair on the last day of school? She wasn't angry, just mystified while pointing to the "board tooth" I had filled. Her other hand contained a small shiny filling in it. It turned out that the amalgam board filling had indeed fatally fractured internally when smashed by the board examiner, but managed to stay together long enough for me to pass. I had gotten lucky. I wonder how many other students got the shaft from his "smashing" grading routine? I apologized again to the patient, replaced the broken filling, dismissed her, and sat down to think. It was rare for me to be in a zoned-out, introspective state. Nevertheless, there I sat, staring into space, in deep contemplation. Dentistry suddenly appeared scary; it appeared to be a profession of profound frustrations and constant/endless, unavoidable failures. Was this what I signed up for? Were the boards merely a cynical rebuke to four years of optimism? Could I handle dentistry as a career? Obviously, dentists out there did, and some weren't alcoholics or suicidal. I snapped out of my trance upon being poked by Dr. J., a beloved and benevolent module instructor/

director. He sympathized with my momentary pain and prophetically said, "You'll be all right, just take it day by day." That sounded to me like an AA soliloquy; I think it came from personal experience.

96

What Killed Dr. J.?

Dr. J. was long retired from private practice and was
the chief dental instructor/director of our senior module
practice. He was actually more than that: mentor, confidante,
humorist, and teacher. But, his hands shook as if he had
Parkinson's. Did he have some type of neurological disorder?
A persistent rumor kept circulating with each class, namely
that he was slowly succumbing to mercury poisoning. Crap!
Elemental mercury is a large constituent of amalgam fillings.
Did the mercury vapors hurt him? Maybe he handled the
mercury with his bare hands, as old timer dentists frequently
did? Perhaps he poisoned himself without knowing it at
the time? What a terrible way to go downhill, and all from
an occupational hazard. Damn it! He was such a nice guy.
One day before graduation, he and I got to talking and
I flat out asked him about his "mercury" disability. He
looked confused at first, then finally relented and admitted
that he indeed suffered from mercury toxicity, and his
symptoms were worsening. I asked him if we students and

future dentists were risking our health surrounded by this toxic liquid metal all around us? He told me that's what he originally also thought. However, he went on to tell me, rather comically mind you, that it was actually a lifetime of eating tons of tuna fish that did him in. A neurologist told him so. What? It turns out that methyl mercury (the form of mercury found in tuna fish and other large, long-lived fishes) is readily absorbed into the bloodstream, whereas the kind found in amalgam fillings and old thermometers (elemental mercury) is basically not. Perhaps it was a combination of both types of mercury, an overload? I digested his statements and thanked him. Dr. J. passed away a few years after I graduated. Was it really caused by StarKist? I don't know. After all, he was 80. By the way, every time I feed my cat tuna fish, I think of Dr. J. and that dang rumor. What a memory to have!

97

The "Shocking" Award

For four years Rebecca had dismissed me as a fool, an idiot, a dental imposter. At least that's what her friends told me. She was well known to be very serious and studious, with no time for parties, get-togethers or frivolities. She was going to conquer the world of dentistry! Guys like me made no sense and were just in her way. I was the opposite of her, or was I? Her eyes would roll and she would shake her head in utter dismay whenever I had opened my pie-hole to let out a humorous remark or two. I'm sure she wondered what a "comedian" was doing in dental college. An impromptu graduation awards ceremony was set up in the large front foyer of our school, on the last day of class, prior to our very last morning seminar. Some administration wonks had their minions hastily assemble us and proceeded quickly to disburse individual course awards and recognition plaques. I received the Periodontal Award for Excellence, to muted and awkward congratulations. Then the valedictorian got his medal, the salutatorian accepted his ribbon…and I

received a certificate for finishing third in the class! What!!??
Walking toward the school's vice dean to gather my reward,
amongst a bit of clapping and hollering from my closest
friends, I happened to notice Rebecca unashamedly staring
at me, mouth agape, shaking her head and her fists all balled
up. What's *he* doing up there? When did *he* get so smart?
Afterwards during our last seminar in the auditorium, she
kept turning around to look at me in that shocked, quizzical
and questioning sort of way. How did that clown finish so
high up in the class? It just couldn't be, or could it? I was
planning to confront her later on, just to rub it in, and ask
what *her* class rank was. I didn't get the chance, however. She
probably would have socked me really hard. Anyway, never,
ever judge a book by its cover, well, except for this one maybe!

98

No OKU For You!

Can you really blackball a student? I mean, a standout scholarly type that just happens to rub you the wrong way? Apparently, yes! Our four-year class president had managed to anger the higher-ups to such an extent that he was "maliciously" denied entry into the national dental honor society Omicron Kappa Upsilon. When the senior prosthodontics professor surreptitiously tiptoed around the senior modules giving us thirteen select men (no women made the cut in our year) the "nod of inclusion," our class president was left out. He was not tapped! He immediately sought an audience with the school dean, but to no avail. No OKU for you! Privately, we debated the astonishing and disturbing situation. Maybe he wasn't good in the labs, maybe he couldn't cut teeth, maybe he missed some clinical requirements to graduate? No maybes. He was the class president and had the highest class average! Come on. He had fought long and hard for us for four years. Administrators, chairmen, professors, and even secretaries all got an earful from him if even a single test question had seemed unfair or improperly graded. Everyone in school knew him. So what better way to douse some of that ardor and *chutzpah?* Deny him the obvious honor, of course! "They" finally got even in the end. It was very embarrassing watching him stoically deliver a very thoughtful valedictory commencement address. The speech had no malice but no joy, either. He stood there without the special gold braids that adorned we OKU members; we all knew what he was missing. Rumor had it that he eventually specialized in oral surgery. Maybe his hands weren't that good after all? Still, to deny the class valedictorian an obvious honor was reprehensible but, hey, this was PU College of Dentistry!

99

Uncle Fung's

I was on top of the world that Saturday. The graduation festivities were held at a popular town hall as a special event and it felt good to have my family, in-laws and wife partake in them with me. My mother was beaming. My father looked proud, I think. My wife wouldn't let go of my arm! This was her prize as well as mine. The school even handed out "joke" spouse certificates in honor of the partners that went through the dental school ringer along with their significant others. Small groups of elated and relieved ex-students and family members could be seen everywhere. Regardless, after all the speeches, faux glad-handing and wild promises to keep in touch, our class slowly dispersed, like an ink spot in a glass of water. However, you could still pick out the doctoral caps and gowns of the new dentists in the distance as they slowly faded from view and my dental life. I also kept my attire on for a good while, my badge of courage. Now it was time to feast and celebrate. Fortunately, my wife had made reservations at a locally fantastic Chinese eatery called Uncle Fung's. It was a classic and classy establishment in the middle of the busy town. Our familial entourage headed that way slowly, still encountering recent grads along our route. All my future plans were suspended for a day; it was refreshing to relax and soak in the joyous occasion. I had recently taken the dental board exams successfully and gotten into one of the country's very best dental residency programs. And I had re-signed our lease to keep us living in that same apartment; no moving. Yeah, I was happy! Now it was time to eat. We arrived early, well, early by some restaurant standards, I guess. It was 1 p.m. when I opened the front door to enter Uncle Fung's. We looked around and saw white apron-clothed Asian bodies littered about the spacious foyer, sleeping on couches, futons and on the floor! They all jolted upright and stared at us foreigners as we questioningly stared back. Were they open for lunch? What about that reservation? The nimble manager appeared out of nowhere, apologized profusely in broken Mandarin, and quickly ushered us into a private banquet room, just for our family. Nevertheless, I couldn't help but wonder about all those "employees." Had it been a late night before? Were they hung over, or still drunk? Did they just get off the boat and were exhausted? Did they live inside the restaurant, as illegal sublet tenants? I knew something about that! All those questions; no answers. Once they shook off their slumbers, these polite "workers" rapidly started catering to us. No English was spoken. Tsing Tao beer all around in many rounds, and unbelievable Chinese food on three large Lazy Susans in the middle of a spacious table. We were impressed with the spreads and the super service. It was the first time my parents had tasted Chinese cuisine and were blown away. Perhaps it was all the beer, or the General Tsao's chicken and moo goo gai pan. Anyway, all family members had a good time and we left, full and satisfied. It had been a memorable day. Four years of hard work and deprivation culminated in a graduation, a party and a fortune cookie. I never did read my fortune. Maybe I should have.

Take a powder!

100

Disclaimer For Dentists

To any dentist who just happened to mistakenly read this book in the bathroom before using it as kindling: you know what I'm talking about. We all suffer a bit from that ongoing dreaded disease called Aggravation Saturation; it started on the first day of class and never let up.

I sincerely hope you will have, or have had, a long and satisfying career in dentistry. After selling my last practice, I have worked part time as a commissioned employee-dentist in various offices and continue to "hustle" for the legal tender. Do I miss ownership? Not on your Nellie! Regardless, I am truly grateful for having had the opportunity to learn and practice dentistry, as a specialist, and earn a good income from it. Nevertheless, it may finally be time to step off the dental merry-go-round and stop the stresses. But complete retirement? Nah! Who says you can't teach an old *putz* at least one new trick. Is it too late to become an entomologist? Never say never!

Was all that dental school "fun" worth it? It's hard to tell; it could have gone either way.

101

Disclaimer For Students

To any prospective dental student having read this book as gospel and still wondering if a dental career is feasible: if you can stomach the following axioms, you will most likely succeed.

1. "Today's hero is tomorrow's goat."
2. "Most patients will turn on you in a second."
3. "Don't expect gratitude or payment."

Having read this book and the above, you may be thinking that after graduating from dental school I became overly cynical and harsh, and perhaps you are correct. On the other hand, perhaps a career spent being the brunt of inhumane behavior warped me, somewhat. Perhaps somebody should have given me salient inside information before I decided on a career in dentistry. Perhaps, perhaps, perhaps... Forewarned is forearmed! You decide.

Hurray! You succeeded in getting admitted to and finally graduating from dental college. Now comes a career filled with unrealistic expectations, unwarranted malpractice suits, pro bono work (unintentional, of course), high stress and aggravation saturation. Maybe you should have become an entomologist, instead? You decide.

Lease the obligatory Beemer or Benz, marry a trophy wife/husband, buy a couple of vacation homes in the Caribbean, build a huge practice or two, have kids, and be grateful and happy. I drive a Hyundai, but own six cars. I married a *hottie blondie* pharmacist who is long retired and still looks hot in her birthday suit at our Bahamas beachfront vacation villa. I've had my dental day in the sun and sold three successful practices. And I'm still paying college tuitions; all those Ivies are damn expensive! I am very grateful; am I happy, though? You decide.

Good luck.

102

Last Words

Dental school: A motley crew of mostly naïve and studious perfectionists molded into oral caregivers expecting gratitude and compensation from an indifferent and imperfect, yet demanding, public.

Was all the mental anguish, high tuition and sacrifice required for dental school worth it? Were my best intentions of dentally helping and healing humanity realized? Probably, but I'm not completely sure. I sometimes ponder those very questions as I gratefully peer out at the ocean from my *other* seaside vacation villa on the Baja peninsula, in Mexico. However the jury is still out– thirty-plus years and counting. Entomology may still be an option!

Thanks for the read.

About the Author

Dr. I. Mayputz (not his real name) graduated with highest honors from high school, from pharmacy college and summa cum laude from dental school. After completing a master's degree in prosthodontics at a then prestigious institution, he embarked on his dental career in private practice. He once briefly toyed with the idea of earning a Ph.D. to become an actual entomologist, but ultimately decided on a dreadfully stressful albeit lucrative career, instead. In addition to being an elite master's athlete, author, naturalist and part-time naturist, he is also known as a caustic wit and provocateur. He wrote this book to entertain family, friends, and any curious sod willing to peek behind the dental curtain.

For more alleged levity, please read
Pharmacy College: Crazy Daze and Hazy Nites
By Dr. I. Mayputz.
Mr. Nick Productions, LLC., ©2017

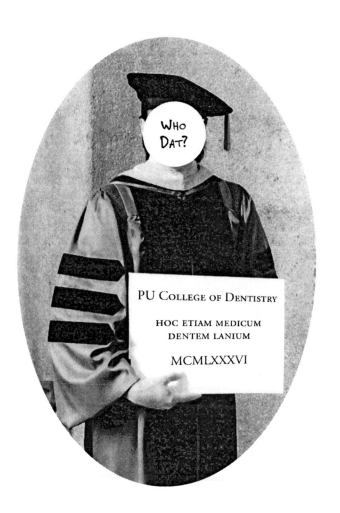